ECG for Beginners

Anandaraja Subramanian
MD DM FCE

Consultant
Department of Cardiology
Indira Gandhi Government General Hospital and
Postgraduate Institute
Puducherry, India

Raja J Selvaraj
MD DNB FCE

Associate Professor
Department of Cardiology
Jawaharlal Institute of Postgraduate Medical
Education and Research
Puducherry, India

The Health Sciences Publisher

New Delhi | London | Philadelphia | Panama

Jaypee Brothers Medical Publishers (P) Ltd.

Headquarters

Jaypee Brothers Medical Publishers (P) Ltd.
4838/24, Ansari Road, Daryaganj
New Delhi 110 002, India
Phone: +91-11-43574357
Fax: +91-11-43574314
E-mail: jaypee@jaypeebrothers.com

Overseas Offices

J.P. Medical Ltd.
83, Victoria Street, London
SW1H 0HW (UK)
Phone: +44 20 3170 8910
Fax: +44 (0)20 3008 6180
E-mail: info@jpmedpub.com

Jaypee-Highlights Medical Publishers Inc.
City of Knowledge, Bld. 237, Clayton
Panama City, Panama
Phone: +1 507-301-0496
Fax: +1 507-301-0499
E-mail: cservice@jphmedical.com

Jaypee Medical Inc.
The Bourse
111, South Independence Mall East
Suite 835, Philadelphia, PA 19106, USA
Phone: +1 267-519-9789
E-mail: jpmed.us@gmail.com

Jaypee Brothers Medical Publishers (P) Ltd.
17/1-B, Babar Road, Block-B, Shaymali
Mohammadpur, Dhaka-1207
Bangladesh
Mobile: +08801912003485
E-mail: jaypeedhaka@gmail.com

Jaypee Brothers Medical Publishers (P) Ltd.
Bhotahity, Kathmandu, Nepal
Phone: +977-9741283608
E-mail: Kathmandu@jaypeebrothers.com

Website: www.jaypeebrothers.com
Website: www.jaypeedigital.com

ECG for Beginners

First Edition: **2015**

ISBN 978-93-5152-660-5

Printed at Rajkamal Electric Press, Plot No. 2, Phase-IV, Kundli, Haryana.

ECG for Beginners

Preface

Interpretation of ECG can be intimidated for beginners. Though many books are available on this subject, there are none which highlight the concepts in interpretation with practical examples. Our idea is to give a practical example with case history for each of the possible abnormalities in the ECG. This way, the beginner will know what to concentrate on in a given clinical setting, instead of getting lost in the whole ECG. We have assembled a unique set of ECGs, each one to teach a particular abnormality. Some of the ECGs with multiple abnormalities are repeated to teach different concepts. Also, we have simplified the subject keeping in mind the beginner's aptitude. The book is specifically intended for the beginners: students (Medical, Nursing and Allied Medical Professionals), first year postgraduates (Medicine, Anesthesia, Pediatrics) and practicing physicians. The book is not a complete ECG textbook. Each chapter will have a brief text on a particular concept followed by practical examples. The synopsis section summarizes all concepts in a very simple manner. An appendix is added which will give more information on a given abnormality seen in the ECG. We hope the readers will learn immensely from this unique format.

Anandaraja Subramanian
Raja J Selvaraj

Contents

1

Basics of ECG

Electrocardiogram (ECG) is the recording of the electrical activity of the heart on a graph paper. The electrical activity is generated by the activation (depolarization) and inactivation (repolarization) of the atrial and the ventricular muscle (myocardium). The myocardium is activated by the conduction system of the heart. The electrical activity of the conduction system is itself too small to be recorded by the ECG! ECG machine is a modified galvanometer that outputs the electrical activity of the heart in the form of tracings. The machine is normally standardized to output one millivolt of electrical activity as 10 millimeter deflection along the vertical axis of the graph paper (Figure 1.1). The standard speed of the paper is 25 mm/sec.

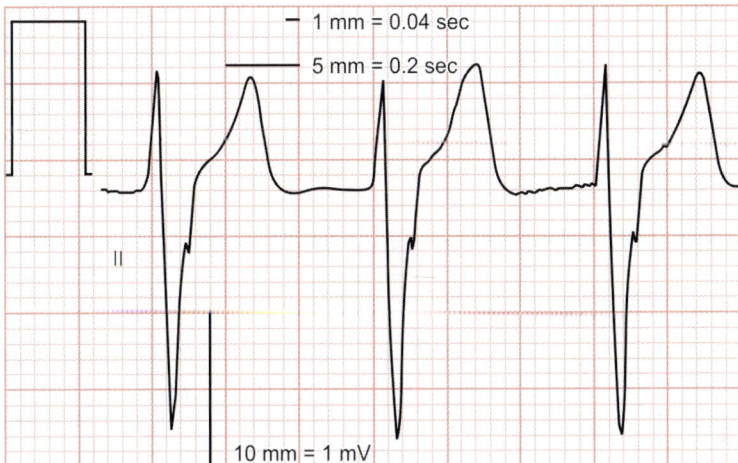

Figure 1.1 Standard calibration of ECG

■ CONDUCTION SYSTEM OF THE HEART

The conduction system of the heart consists of the sinoatrial node (SA node), preferential interatrial conduction fibers, atrioventricular node (AV node), bundle of His, bundle branches (right and left), and the Purkinje network (Figure 1.2). The left bundle divides into two fascicles (anterosuperior and posteroinferior) before ramification into the Purkinje network. Any of the cells in the conduction system is capable of spontaneous firing and initiating the heartbeat. The SA node is the normal pacemaker of the heart and impulse originating from it activates the rest of the heart. Under normal conditions, the frequency of depolarization of the SA node is faster, and so it overrides the other foci in the conduction system. However, when the SA node is diseased, other subsidiary pacemakers can take over the rhythm of the heart.

Impulses originating from the SA node activate the atria, with the right atrium being activated first, followed by the left atrium. The impulse also travels towards the AV node by preferential conduction pathways formed by the atrial musculature. Once the impulse reaches the AV node, there is a delay due to slowing of conduction in the AV node. From the AV node, the impulse spreads to the bundle

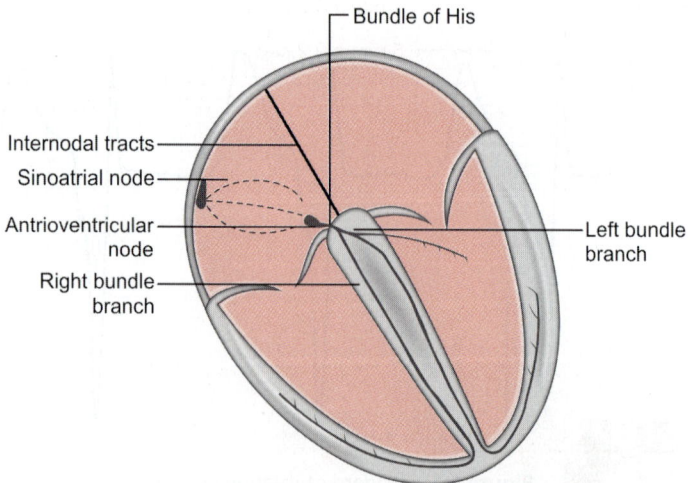

Figure 1.2 The conduction system of the heart

of His, the bundle branches and the fascicles. Finally, the impulse reaches the Purkinje fibers in the endocardium of the heart. The impulse reaches the endocardium of all regions of the heart near simultaneously and results in synchronized depolarization of the entire ventricular myocardium.

Leads

For recording the electrical activity, electrode pairs called leads are used. Each of these electrode pairs (leads) will record the electrical activity of the heart as seen by them. It is true that the more the number of leads we use, the more complete picture can be obtained about the electrical activity of the heart. However, using too many leads will be cumbersome and using less will lead to insufficient data. The standard practice is to use 12 leads to record the heart's electrical activity. Six of these leads record the electrical activity in the frontal plane (limb leads) and six of them record the electrical activity in the horizontal plane (chest leads, Figure 1.3 and Table 1.1). The leads

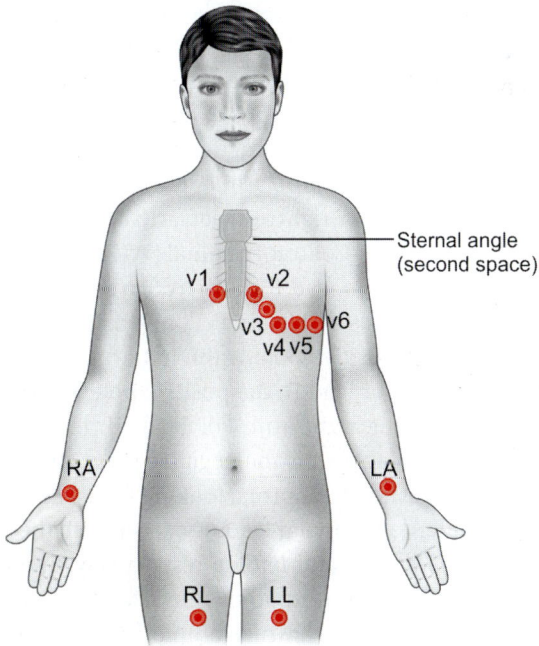

Figure 1.3 Electrode placement for recording ECG

Table 1.1 Derivation of the leads from the electrodes (see Figure 1.3)

Lead label	Negative	Positive
I	RA	LA
II	RA	LL
III	LA	RL
aVR	RA	*WCT
aVL	LA	*WCT
aVF	LL	*WCT
V1	V1	WCT
V2	V2	WCT
V3	V3	WCT
V4	V4	WCT
V5	V5	WCT
V6	V6	WCT

WCT – Wilson's Central Terminal
* WCT is modified by removing the corresponding active electrode

can be bipolar or unipolar. Bipolar leads record the electrical activity between two active electrodes (positive and negative), while the unipolar leads record the electrical activity between an active and an inactive electrode. For the unipolar recordings, reference electrode is formed by connecting the right arm, left arm and left leg electrodes together to form a Wilson Central Terminal (WCT).

The limb leads include lead I, II, III, aVR, aVL and aVF. Leads I, II and III are bipolar leads and leads aVR, aVL and aVF are unipolar leads. For lead I, the positive pole is the left arm and the negative pole is the right arm. For lead II, the positive pole is the left leg and the negative pole is the right arm. For lead III, the left leg is the positive pole and the left arm is the negative pole. Misplacement of the electrodes can result in abnormal looking ECGs! Leads aVR, aVL and aVF are augmented unipolar leads recorded with the active pole on the right arm, left arm and left leg respectively. The indifferent electrode for these leads is formed by removing the corresponding active electrode from the WCT, which amplifies the signal by 50%.

The six chest leads include V1 to V6 and all are unipolar leads. It is important to place the chest leads in standard positions to make a meaningful interpretation of the ECG. V1 is positioned in the right fourth intercostal space adjacent to the sternum and V2 is placed in the left fourth intercostal space adjacent to the sternal border. Next V4 is placed in the fifth intercostal space in the midclavicular line. V3 is placed midway between V2 and V4. V5 is placed in the anterior axillary line along the same line as V4 and V6 is place in the mid-axillary line along the same line as V4 and V5.

In addition to these 12 leads, special leads are sometimes used for recording activity from the atria, right ventricle and posterior side of the heart. Normal ECG tracing consists of waves, intervals and segments. The waves include P, QRS, T and U. The intervals include PR and QT intervals. The segments include PR and ST segments. Each of them will be addressed in subsequent chapters.

Uses

The ECG can be used to diagnose coronary artery disease, chamber enlargements, arrhythmias, inherited electrical disorders, drug toxicities and electrolyte imbalances. Each of these conditions affects the activation (depolarization) or inactivation (repolarization) of the heart and thus gives an indirect clue to their presence. Since ECG is not a direct measure of any of these abnormalities except for some arrhythmias, their use in these conditions is not fool proof. Therefore, there can be false negatives and false positives. Despite this, ECG is immensely helpful as an initial investigation in these conditions. As with any investigation, the significance of an abnormal finding has to be considered along with the total clinical picture. ECG being inexpensive, noninvasive and widely available, basic knowledge of the same will benefit the practicing primary care physician.

2   **Heart Rate**

The ECG can be used to readily calculate the heart rate. ECG records the atrial and ventricular activity during each cardiac cycle. The atrial activity is represented by the P wave and the ventricular activity by the QRS complex in the ECG. The pulse, which we feel by palpating the arteries, is generated by the ventricular activity (contraction). Thus, by determining the rate of ventricular activity on the ECG, we can infer the pulse rate of the subject.

▉ REGULAR RATE

When the rate is regular, we can use a short-cut method. The short-cut method for determining the ventricular rate is to count the number of large or small squares between any two R waves. When we use the large squares, the heart rate is 300 divided by the number of large squares. When using the small squares, the heart rate is 1500 divided by the number of small squares. Alternatively, we can use the method described below for irregular rates also to calculate the heart rate.

▉ IRREGULAR RATE

When the RR intervals are irregular, then one needs a rhythm strip to calculate the heart rate (rhythm strip is recording from one or more leads for prolonged time). Standard 12 lead ECG recordings usually include a rhythm strip either at the bottom or separately. The standard ECG records the electrical activity on a moving graph paper at a standard rate. This rate is normally 25 mm/sec unless specified otherwise. Put simply, 25 mm on the graph paper (ECG paper), which is five large squares, corresponds to one second time period (1000 milliseconds). To calculate the heart rate in case of irregular rhythm, mark a time interval of 6 or 10 seconds on the ECG paper (equal to distance between 30 or 50 large squares respectively). Now simply count the number of QRS complexes (ventricular activity) within that time interval. This gives the number of pulses (ventricular activity) in the 6- or 10-second interval. To obtain the ventricular rate in 60 seconds, multiply this number by 10 or 6 respectively and this gives the heart rate per minute. Note that a standard 12 lead ECG is 25 cm (10 seconds) long.

DERIVATION OF THE SHORT-CUT METHOD

As we discussed earlier, the ECG paper moves at a speed of 25 mm/sec. Therefore, one minute, which is 60 seconds, corresponds to 1500 small squares, or 300 large squares. If there are n large squares between two R waves, there will be $300/n$ R waves in one minute, which gives the pulse rate.

1. A 50-year-old man underwent routine clinical examination and investigations for insurance purposes. His 12 lead ECG is shown below. What is the heart rate?

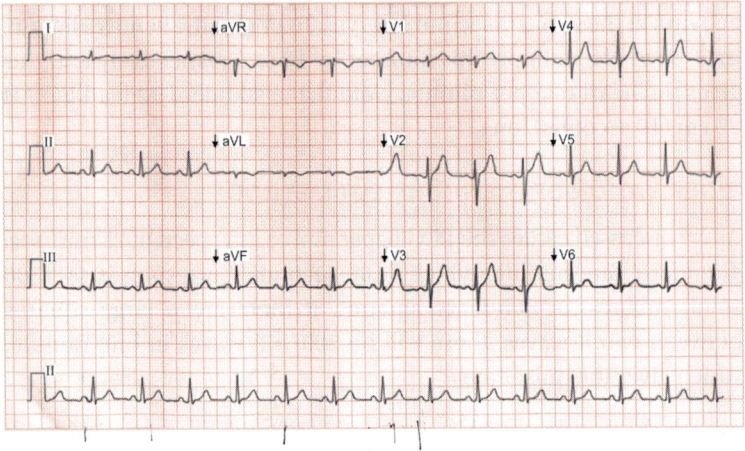

(a) 100
(b) 85
(c) 75
(d) 60

The first step in the calculation of rate is to look at the regularity of the QRS complex. For this, one should look at the rhythm strip shown at the bottom. In the above ECG, the QRS complexes occur at regular intervals. The approximate number of large squares between two consecutive QRS complexes is three-and-a-half (the trick is to select a QRS that falls at the start of the large squares, i.e. thick line of the graph). In this example, complex 3 (arrow) in the rhythm strip falls on the thick line and it is easy to count the large squares from there. Hence, the heart rate is 300/3.5, which is approximately 85. The heart rate is between 60 and 100 beats per minute and so it is normal. If the number of large squares between two QRS complexes is more than 3 (heart rate 100 per minute) or less than 5 (heart rate 60 per minute), the heart rate is normal.

2. A 35-year-old woman presented to the emergency department with a history of sudden onset palpitations for the past two hours. She also complained of giddiness and mild chest discomfort. On examination, the pulse is thready and fast; blood pressure is 100/70 mm Hg. The ECG of the patient is shown below. What is the ventricular rate?

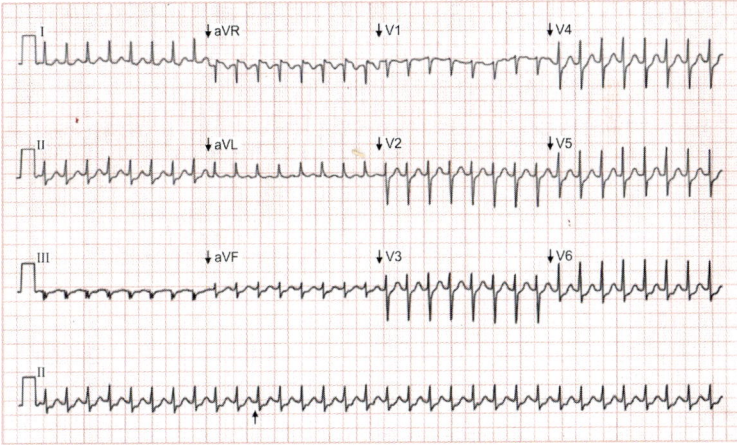

(a) 136
(b) 150
(c) 166
(d) 188

Here again the rate is regular by eyeballing but fast. When the heart rate is high, to minimize the error, it is better to count the small squares. To calculate the heart rate, select the QRS complex that falls on a thick line and start counting the number of small squares. For example, the complex marked by the arrow falls on a thick line and we see there are 8 small squares and so the heart rate is 1500/8, which is approximately 188 per minute. The rate is more than 100 and, hence, indicates tachycardia. There are many causes of tachycardia, including sinus tachycardia, atrial tachycardia, junctional tachycardia and paroxysmal supraventricular tachycardia (PSVT). We will discuss them in later chapters.

3. A 25-year-old woman, known patient of rheumatic heart disease with severe mitral stenosis, presented with acute onset weakness of left upper and lower limbs. CT scan showed a small infarct in the right basal ganglia region. A 12 lead ECG was recorded. What is the heart rate?

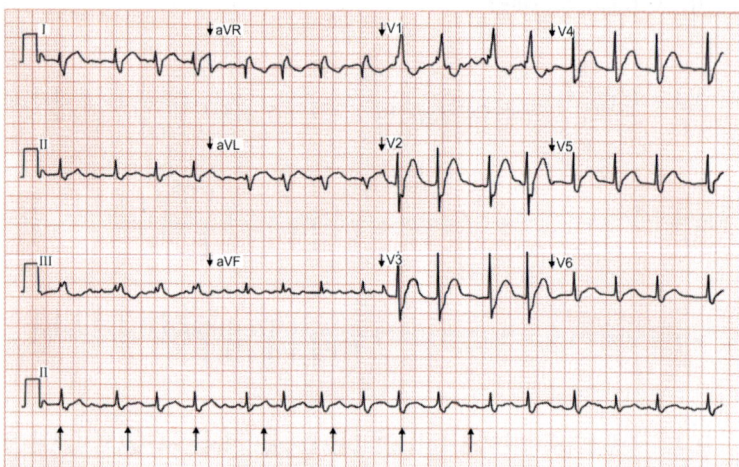

(a) 100
(b) 110
(c) 120
(d) 130

In this ECG, the RR intervals are irregular. Next step is to select a six-second interval (equivalent to 30 large squares). Then simply count the number of QRS complexes in the 6-second interval and multiply that by 10 to give the heart rate. In the ECG shown, the up pointing arrows mark out the time intervals. The time interval between two consecutive arrows is one second. There are 10 QRS complexes in six seconds and so the heart rate is 100 per minute. Alternately, one can use a 10-second interval and multiply the number of QRS complexes by six to get the heart rate. Using longer time intervals decreases the error of calculation. Causes of fast heart rates with irregular rhythm include atrial fibrillation, atrial flutter, and multifocal atrial tachycardia. We will discuss them in later chapters.

4. A 67-year-old man reported to his physician with recurrent episodes of giddiness and one episode of syncope. He is not on any medications. What is his approximate heart rate based on the ECG shown below?

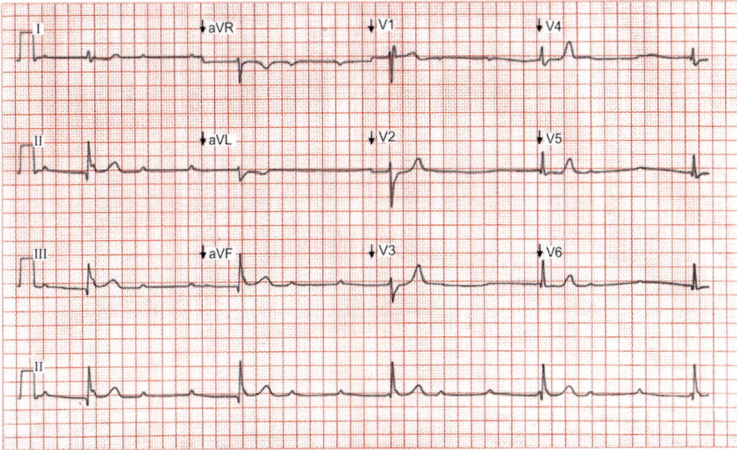

(a) 27
(b) 40
(c) 55
(d) 36

In this ECG, the QRS complexes are regular and there are approximately 11 large squares between two QRS complexes. Application of the method described earlier gives us a heart rate of approximately 27/min. The rate is lower than 60 and, hence, it is bradycardia (slow heart rate). Causes of bradycardia include sinus bradycardia, junctional rhythm, and atrioventricular blocks. We will discuss them in later chapters.

5. A 45-year-old man was admitted to the cardiac intensive care unit for acute inferior wall myocardial infarction. He was noticed to have irregular heartbeat by the nurse and this was confirmed in the ECG tracings of his monitor. A 12 lead ECG was done. What are the atrial and ventricular rates as calculated from the ECG?

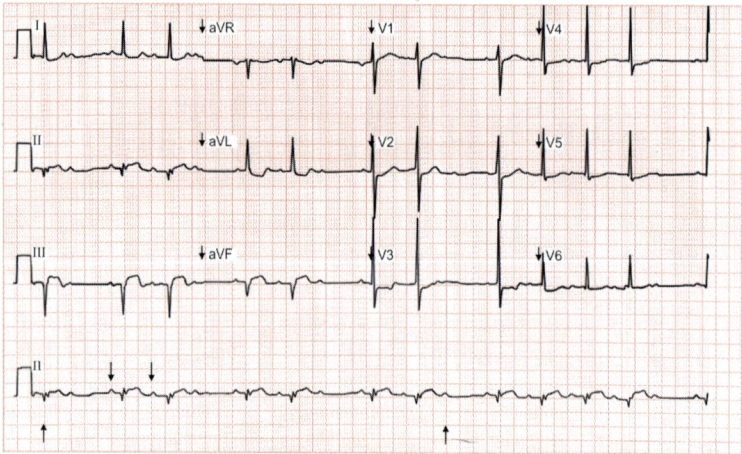

(a) 100 and 70
(b) 70 and 100
(c) 80 and 90
(d) 90 and 80

We can calculate the atrial and ventricular rates separately from the ECG. Normally, there is one-to-one relation between the atrial activity (P wave) and ventricular activity (QRS complex). However, there can be situations where this association is lost. In such situations, it is better to report the atrial and ventricular rates separately. The method is the same as described earlier. We have to consider the P waves to calculate the atrial rate and the QRS complexes to calculate the ventricular rate. In the ECG shown, the P waves occur at regular intervals and there are three large squares between two P waves (marked by down-pointing arrows in rhythm strip). The atrial rate is, therefore, 100 per minute. The QRS complexes occur at irregular intervals. So, here a 6-second interval is marked by the up-pointing arrows. There are seven QRS complexes in that interval and so the ventricular rate is 70 per minute.

3

P Wave

The P waves on the ECG represent right and left atrial activation (voltage changes produced by the atria during depolarization). The initial part represents activation of the right atrium and the terminal part represents activation of the left atrium. The mid-part represents overlapping of both left and right atrial activation.

Though we have 12 leads recording this activity, we need to focus only on two leads to understand the normal atrial activation (P wave). These leads are lead II and V1. The normal direction of activation of the atria in the frontal plane is from right superior to left inferior. This occurs along the direction of lead II. Thus, the P wave will be recorded as a positive deflection in lead II. This direction is away from lead aVR and so it will record a negative P wave. The P wave normally has a smooth contour. Abnormal P waves can have a peaked or notched appearance in lead II and may be inverted also. Inverted P waves indicate activation proceeding from low to high right atrium (reverse of normal). In the horizontal plane, the direction of activation is initially anterior and then posterior. Thus, in lead V1, the P wave will be biphasic with an initial positive and a terminal negative deflection.

The normal atria generate a certain amount of electrical activity for a certain amount of time during their activation. The amount of electricity is measured in terms of millivolts (amplitude of the P wave from baseline measured in millimeters). The duration of the activity is measured in terms of milliseconds (duration of the P wave). Enlarged or diseased atria will generate abnormal amount of electricity. Hence, we should know about the normal range of the P wave amplitude and duration in lead II and V1. In lead II, the upper limit of normal P wave amplitude is 2.5 mm (two-and-a-half small squares, 0.25 mV) and upper limit of normal duration is 2.5 mm (two-and-a-half small squares, 100 ms). The upper limit of normal P wave positive deflection in lead V1 is 1.5 mm. The upper limit of terminal negative deflection and duration in lead V1 normally is 1 mm and 0.04 s respectively. Right atrial enlargement results in increased amplitude of the P wave while the left atrial enlargement results in a wider P wave, often with notching in lead II.

1. A 35-year-old man was evaluated for atypical chest pain. What is the abnormality of the P wave?

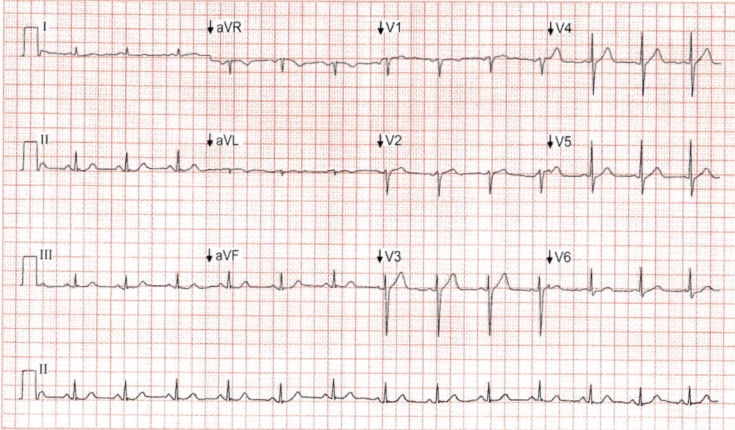

(a) P waves are normal
(b) P waves are wide
(c) P waves are tall
(d) P waves are notched

To comment on the P waves, we have to look at leads II and V1 mainly. The P waves are upright and rounded in lead II. The amplitude and duration of the P waves in these two leads are within the normal range. Though the P wave is not exactly biphasic in lead V1, the overall pattern is within the normal limits. Variations occur secondary to lead placement positions and body habitus. The P waves are positive in lead I. This indicates right to left activation of the atria. Also the P waves are upright in leads II, III and aVF. This indicates that the atria are getting activated in a high-to-low pattern. This is the normal activation pattern of the atria from the sinus node, which is located high in the right atrium.

2. A 30-year-old lady with rheumatic heart disease and severe mitral stenosis was seen in the emergency room for pricking right sided chest pain. What is the abnormality of the P wave ?

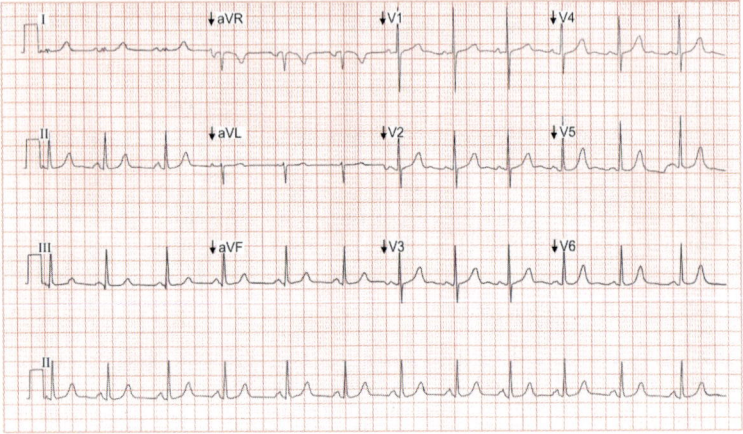

(a) P waves are normal
(b) P waves are wide
(c) P waves are tall
(d) P waves are inverted

Again looking at leads II and V1, we find that the P wave in lead II has a peaked contour and, on close inspection, there is a notch in the P wave. The duration of the P wave is approximately three-and-a-half small squares, which is abnormal. The amplitude of the P wave is less than 2.5 mm. In lead V1, there is only a positive deflection and it is less than 1.5 mm. Thus, the only abnormality in the P wave is the abnormal duration (wide). Wide P waves are commonly seen in case of left atrial enlargement. Wide P waves are also seen whenever there is intra-atrial conduction delay that leads to slow conduction in the atria. Intra-atrial conduction delay occurs with diseased and fibrotic atria. The case vignette suggests left atrial enlargement secondary to mitral stenosis as the cause of wide P wave.

3. A 67-year-old man, chronic smoker, presented with breathlessness to the emergency. What is the abnormality of the P waves in the ECG?

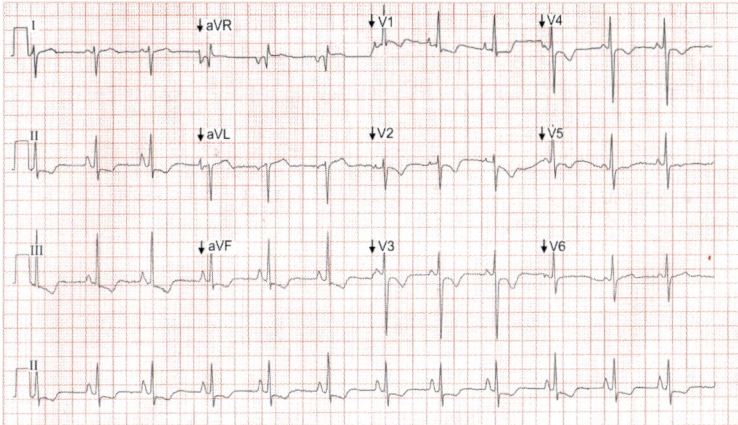

(a) P waves are normal
(b) P waves are wide
(c) P waves are tall
(d) P waves are notched

The striking abnormality is that the P waves are tall in lead II (>2.5 mm) and V1 (>1.5 mm). This is an example of abnormal P waves that are tall. This type of P wave is also called as "P Pulmonale". Tall P waves are seen in patients with right atrial enlargement. Causes of right atrial enlargement include tricuspid stenosis, tricuspid regurgitation, pulmonary hypertension from any cause, pulmonary stenosis, etc. The patient is a chronic smoker. The cause of right atrial enlargement in this patient is possibly pulmonary artery hypertension secondary to chronic obstructive airways disease.

4. A 23-year-old woman was detected to have a mid-diastolic murmur at the apex with loud first heart sound and pansystolic murmur at the tricuspid area during routine antenatal visit. What is the P wave abnormality in the ECG?

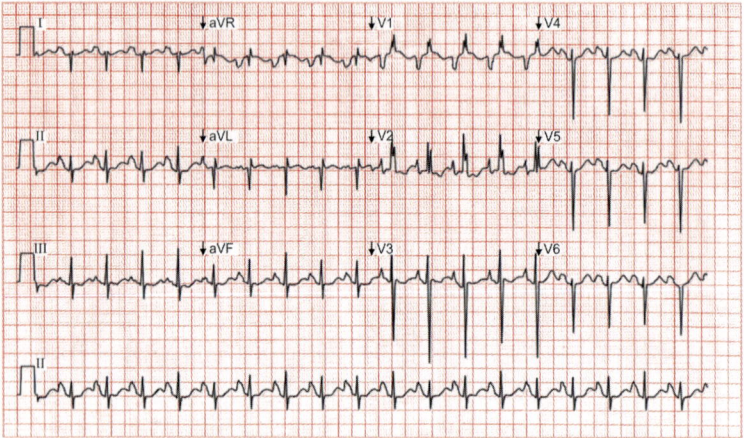

(a) P waves are normal
(b) P waves are wide
(c) P waves are tall
(d) P waves are wide and tall

In this case, the P waves are both tall and wide. Tall and wide P waves are seen with enlargement of both the right and left atria. Biatrial enlargement is seen with cardiomyopathies and left-sided heart disease, leading to pulmonary hypertension.

5. A 26-year-old lady was admitted for right-sided hemiplegia. Cardiovascular evaluation was suggestive of mitral stenosis. What is the P wave abnormality seen in the ECG?

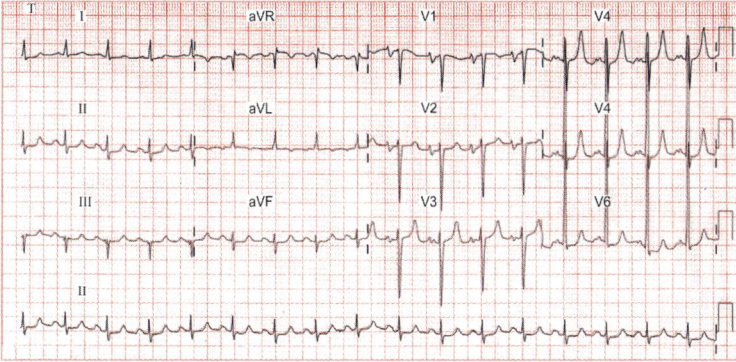

(a) P waves are normal
(b) P waves are notched
(c) P waves are tall
(d) P waves are inverted

The abnormality seen in the ECG is notched P waves. It is clearly seen in lead V4. The second half of the P wave in lead V1 is deep. This is suggestive of left atrial enlargement. Left atrial enlargement is seen with mitral stenosis, mitral regurgitation and left ventricular dysfunction.

6. A 50-year-old lady was evaluated for fitness for gynecological surgery. The treating physician noticed some abnormality in the ECG and requested for cardiologist opinion. What is the abnormality of the P wave?

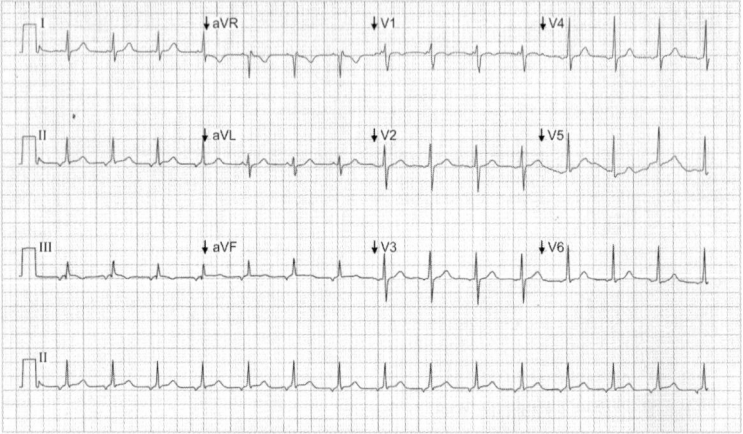

(a) P waves are notched
(b) P waves are tall
(c) P waves are wide
(d) P waves are inverted

The P waves are inverted in inferior leads (leads II, III and aVF). Normally the P waves are upright in inferior leads because the direction of depolarization of the atria are from superior to inferior direction. Inverted P waves indicate that the activation of the atria is occurring from inferior to superior direction. This can happen with low atrial rhythm and junctional rhythms.

7. A 68-year-old man, known case of diabetes and hypertension, presented to the emergency with history of palpitations and giddiness of one-hour duration. What is the abnormality of the P wave in the ECG?

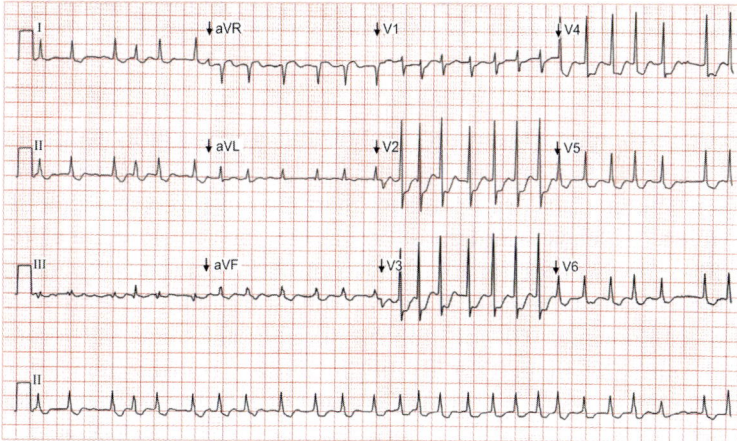

(a) P waves are tall
(b) P waves are normal
(c) P waves are absent
(d) P waves are inverted

In this ECG, one cannot identify a definite P wave. The P waves are absent. Also the rate is fast and rhythm is irregular, which is suggestive of atrial fibrillation. In atrial fibrillation, there is chaotic atrial activity, which may or may not be recorded on the surface ECG. More commonly there will be irregular waves seen as baseline undulations in atrial fibrillation (f-waves). P waves will also be absent in case of sinus node dysfunction and atrial standstill.

4   QRS Complex

The QRS complex is the recording of electricity produced by activation of the ventricular myocardium. 'Q' refers to the first negative wave, 'R' to the first positive wave and 'S' to the negative wave after 'R'. While all 12 leads record the QRS complex, the configuration of the QRS complex varies from one lead to another. Some leads record all the three components (Q, R and S), while some of them record only two components (QR, qR, RS, rS, Rs) and still some will record only one component (Q or R). The difference in configuration is due to the difference in orientation of the 12 leads. Irrespective of the number of components seen, all of them are generally referred to as QRS complex. Q waves are normally seen in lead III and lead aVR. Presence of any Q wave is abnormal in leads V1–V3. Q waves of more than one small square are abnormal in other leads.

The normal duration of the QRS complex is 80–100 ms (two to two-and-half small squares). One has to consider all the twelve leads in measuring the duration of the QRS complex. Amplitude of the QRS is measured from the peak (R wave) to the nadir (q or S wave) of the complex. Normally, the amplitude of the QRS complex is more than 5 mm in the limb leads and more than 10 mm in the chest leads. Values less than this are abnormal. There is no cut-off level for upper limit of QRS voltage. It varies with age, build of subject and myocardial mass. It has to be seen in the clinical context and we will discuss more about QRS voltages in a later chapter (Chamber Enlargement). In the precordial leads, the QRS complex shows progression. Beginning with a small R wave and deep S wave, there is a gradual increase in R wave amplitude and decrease in S wave amplitude from V1–V6. Leads V3 or V4 may record complexes with equal amplitude of R and S waves (equiphasic complex). Prominent R in lead V1 or V2 is called early progression. Absence of equiphasic complex by lead V4 is called late progression.

Normally, the QRS is inscribed as smooth strokes of the individual components. This indicates a rapid spread of depolarization wave and activation of the ventricles by the His-Purkinje fibers. When conduction is not occurring via the Purkinje fibers or when the conduction system is damaged, there will be a delay in the activation of the myocardium. This will be reflected in the ECG by widening of the QRS complex and presence of abnormal notches/slurs in the QRS.

■ CALCULATION OF ELECTRICAL AXIS

During electrical activation of the heart, there is an electric current in all directions produced by the moving activation wavefront. Electrical axis of the heart refers to the mean direction of activation (algebraic sum of all activation) of the heart. We can calculate the mean direction of activation of the atria (P waves) or the ventricles (QRS). Most commonly electrical axis of the ventricles in the frontal plane is calculated. Normally, the mean direction of activation of both the atria and ventricles is from right superior to left inferior in the frontal plane. The 6 leads that are in the frontal plane are I, II, III, aVR, aVL and aVF. These are oriented around the heart forming a hexaxial reference system in the frontal plane. The positive end of lead I (left arm) is designated zero and the negative end 180 degrees. The activation of the heart occurs along the direction of lead II (60 degrees). However, there is considerable variation in the axis and the normal range is from –30 (aVL) to +90 degrees (aVF). Axis between –30 and –90 is called leftward axis and between +90 and +180 is designated as rightward axis. Northwest axis is between +180 and –90 degrees.

A short-cut method to calculate the electrical axis of QRS is to look at leads I and II. If both show predominantly positive QRS, then the axis is normal. If QRS is positive in lead I and negative in lead II, then the axis is leftward. If the QRS is negative in lead I and positive in lead II, then the axis is rightward. If both leads I and II show predominantly negative QRS, then the axis is northwest.

The traditional method is to look for the lead showing equiphasic QRS complex, i.e. waveform showing equal R and S waves or Q and R waves. This means that the activation front is traveling perpendicular to that lead. Now look at the lead perpendicular to it. A predominant positive deflection means the axis is along the positive pole of the lead. The axis will be equal to the designated number assigned to the positive pole. A negative or predominant negative deflection means the axis is towards the negative pole of that lead.

1. A 52-year-old male was seen in the cardiology OPD for occasional episodes of palpitations. ECG taken during this visit is shown. What is the QRS axis?

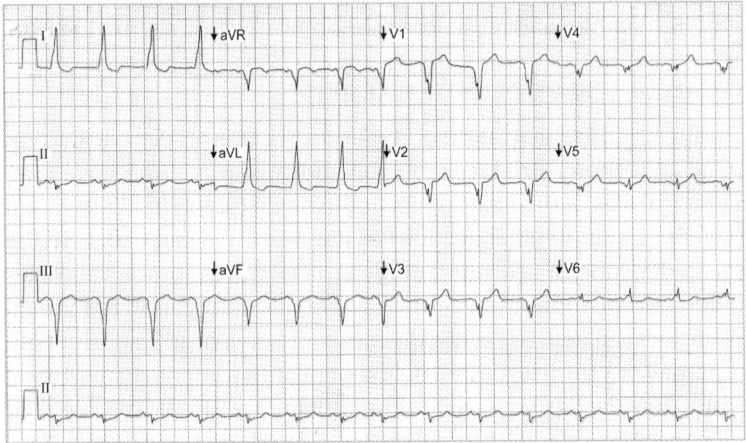

(a) Normal
(b) Leftward
(c) Rightward
(d) Northwest

Here lead I shows a positive QRS deflection and lead II is showing a predominant negative QRS deflection. Based on the short-cut method for calculation of the QRS axis, the axis is leftward. If we apply the traditional method, lead II shows the most equiphasic complex (though more negative), so the QRS vector will be perpendicular to lead II and parallel to lead aVL. Lead aVL shows a positive deflection. So the QRS axis will be around –30 degrees. Hence the QRS axis is leftward.

2. A 40-year-old man was detected to have ECG abnormalities during preoperative work-up. The patient is otherwise asymptomatic. What is the QRS axis in the ECG?

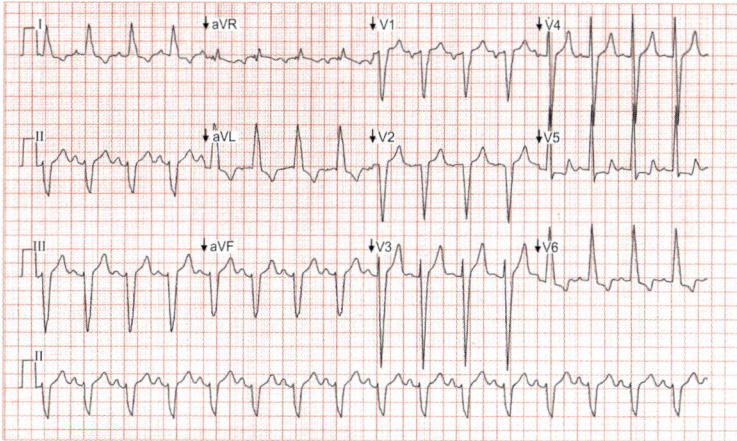

(a) Normal
(b) Leftward
(c) Rightward
(d) Northwest

In this ECG, lead I shows a positive QS complex and lead II shows a negative QRS complex. Hence, by applying the short-cut method, the QRS axis will be leftward.

3. A 48-year-old lady complained of pricking left-sided chest pain of 2 days' duration. She is a diabetic and her elder sister had sustained myocardial infarction. An ECG was obtained. What is the QRS axis?

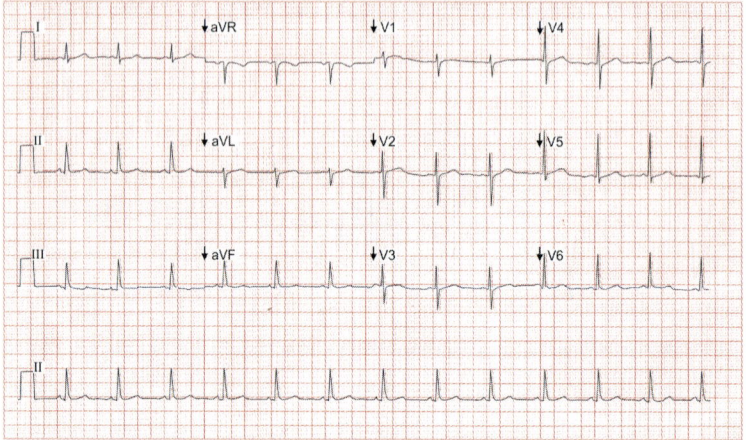

(a) Normal
(b) Leftward
(c) Rightward
(d) Northwest

In this ECG, both lead I and lead II are showing positive QRS complexes. So, the QRS axis is normal.

4. A 12-year-old boy was referred for evaluation of a cardiac murmur. Parents give a history of recurrent respiratory infections in childhood and failure to thrive. An ECG was taken. What is the QRS axis?

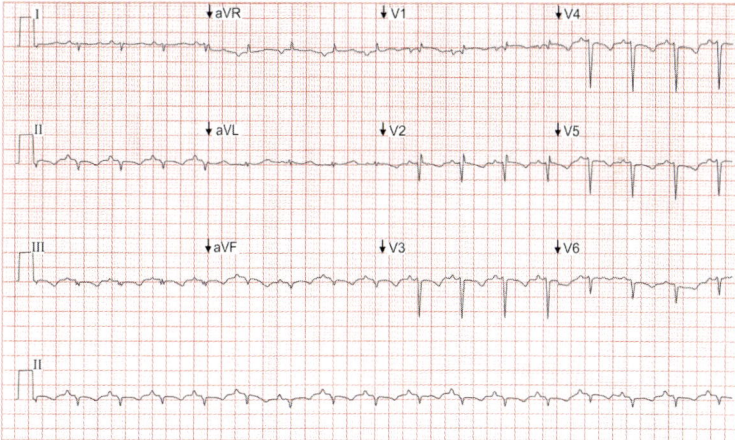

(a) Normal
(b) Leftward
(c) Rightward
(d) Northwest

In this ECG, both the lead I and lead II are showing negative QRS complexes. So, the QRS axis will be northwest.

5. A 50-year-old male underwent 12 lead ECG for the evaluation of atypical chest pain. What is the QRS axis?

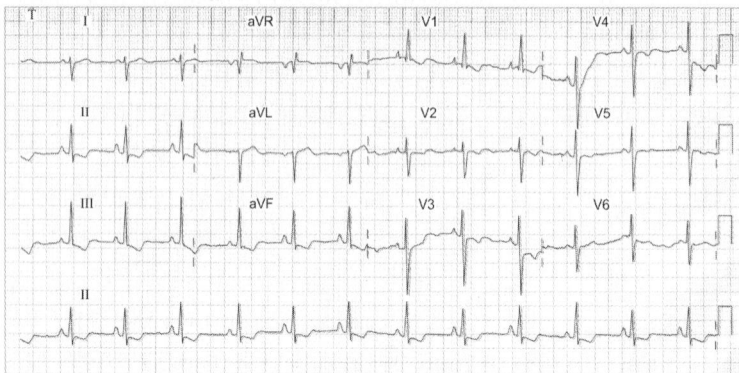

(a) Normal
(b) Leftward
(c) Rightward
(d) Northwest

In this ECG, lead I shows predominant negative deflection and lead II shows positive QRS complex. So, the axis of the QRS will be rightward. If we apply the traditional method, the most equiphasic complex is seen in lead aVR. So, the QRS vector is perpendicular to lead aVR and parallel to lead III. Lead III shows a positive deflection, meaning the vector is traveling towards the positive pole of lead III, which is +120 degrees. Thus, there is right axis deviation of the QRS complex.

6. A 40-year-old man complains of left-sided pricking constant chest pain of 3 days' duration. He smokes two packs of cigarettes a day and his elder brother had undergone coronary artery bypass surgery. Clinical examination was within normal limits. What is the abnormality in the QRS complex?

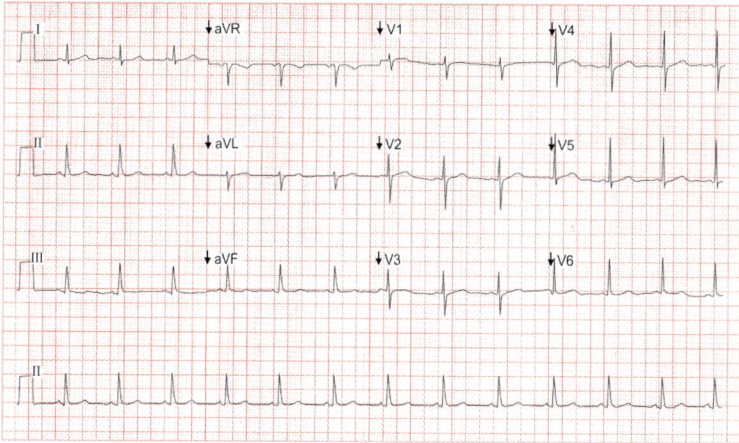

(a) Normal
(b) Wide QRS
(c) Early progression
(d) Late progression

   In the ECG shown the duration of the QRS complex is normal and there is gradual increase in the amplitude of R wave from V1 to V6 indicating normal progression. So the QRS is normal.

7. A 22-year-old lady complains of recurrent episodes of palpitations associated with sweating and giddiness. The episodes terminate spontaneously. A resting 12 lead ECG was recorded. What is the abnormality in the QRS complex?

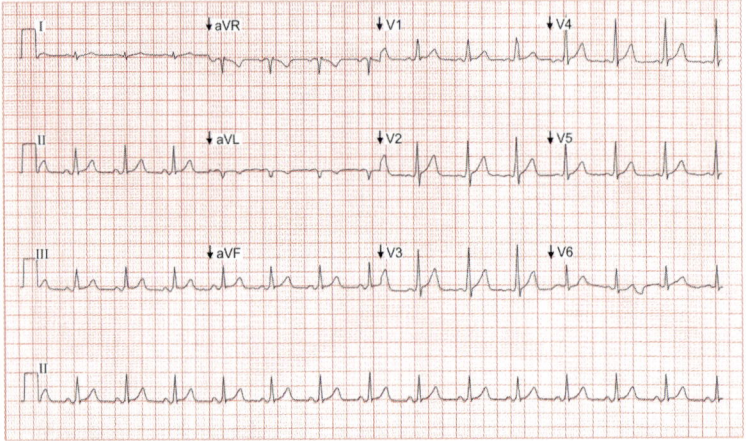

(a)   Normal
(b)   Wide
(c)   Early progression
(d)   Late progression

In this ECG, the QRS complexes in all the precordial leads show a positive deflection starting from lead V1. This is an example of early progression of the QRS complex.

8. A 56-year-old man was admitted to the intensive care unit for acute respiratory infection. He is a heavy smoker with chronic bronchitis. He complained of chest pain and an ECG was recorded. What is the abnormality in the QRS complex?

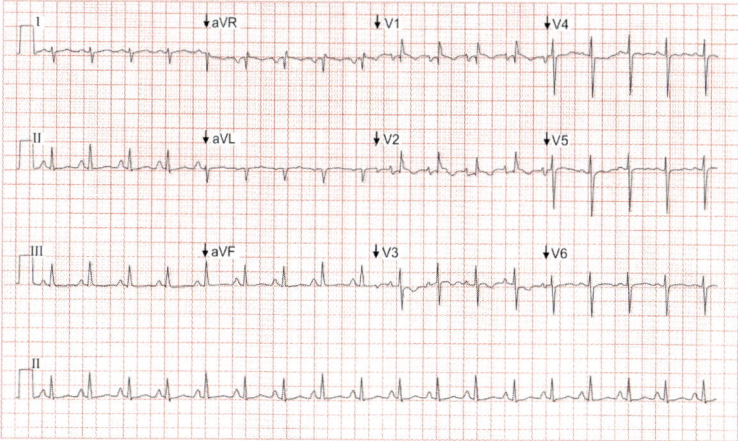

(a) Wide
(b) High amplitude
(c) Early progression
(d) Late progression

In this ECG, again there is predominant positive deflection in lead V1. Therefore, the abnormality seen is early progression.

9. A 64-year-old man complains of breathlessness on exertion for the past 6 months, which has been progressively increasing. Cardiovascular examination was significant for a third heart sound. Chest X-ray showed cardiomegaly. What is the abnormality of the QRS complex in the ECG?

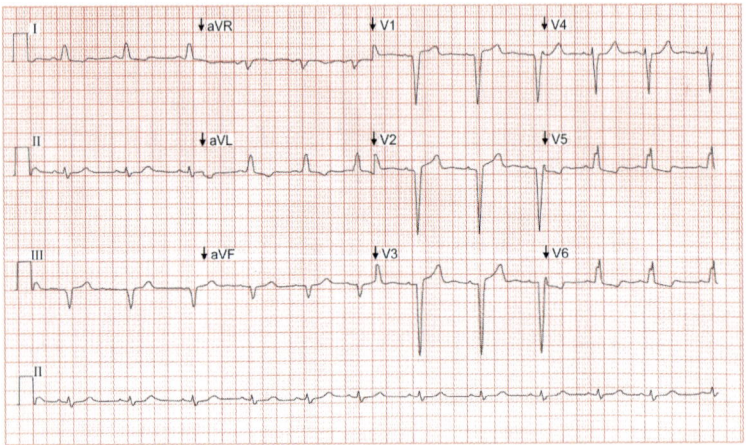

(a) Normal
(b) Low amplitude
(c) Early progression
(d) Late progression

In this ECG, there is predominant R wave of the QRS only in leads V5 and V6. This is an example of late progression of the R wave.

10. A 46-year-old man underwent general health check-up and was noticed to have some abnormality in the ECG. What is the abnormality seen in the QRS complex?

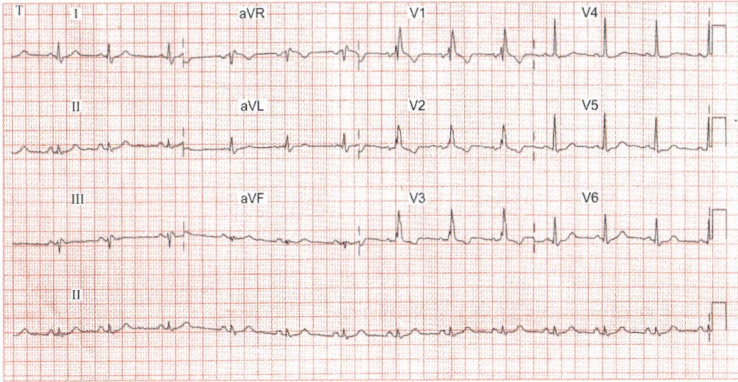

(a) Wide
(b) Wide and notched
(c) Late progression
(d) Low amplitude

The ECG shows QRS complexes that are wide (>120 ms) and are notched, which is better seen in leads V1-V3. QRS complex is produced by activation of the ventricles. Normal activation of the ventricles occurs by way of the His-Purkinje system (HPS). The conduction is very fast in the HPS and results in a normal (narrow) QRS complex. When there is conduction delay in HPS or abnormal activation of the ventricles, the QRS will be prolonged (wide) and will show notches.

11. A 45-year-old man was admitted in the ICU for palpitations and giddiness. The ECG showed tachycardia. The blood pressure was 80 mm of Hg and so he was given DC shock. What is the abnormality of the QRS in the ECG?

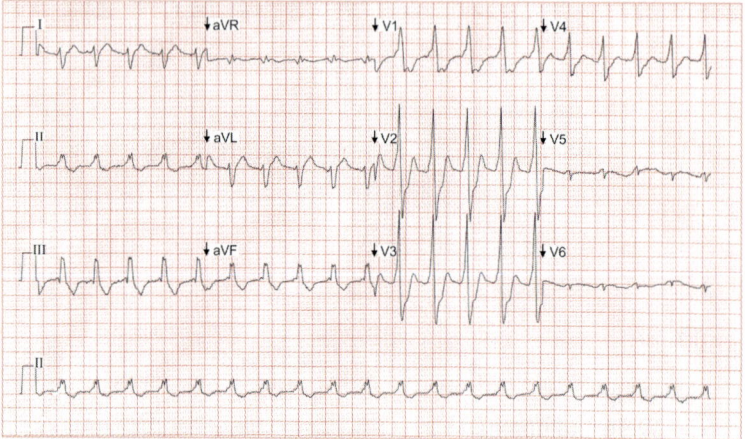

(a) Wide
(b) Low amplitude
(c) Late progression
(d) Leftward axis

The ECG shows wide QRS complexes. The total duration of the QRS complex is more than 120 ms.

12. A 50-year-old lady was seen in the cardiac clinic for exertional angina of 2 weeks' duration. She had suffered from myocardial infarction in the past and was stable on medications earlier. What is the abnormality seen in the QRS complex?

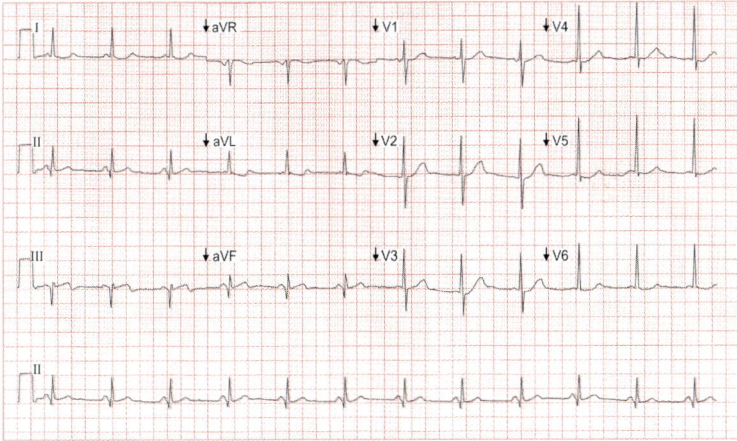

(a) Wide
(b) Low amplitude
(c) Abnormal Q wave
(d) Rightward axis

The ECG shows deep Q waves in leads III and aVF (contiguous leads). Such deep Q waves exceeding 25% of the amplitude of the R wave are abnormal, especially when present in two contiguous leads.

13. A 25-year-old asymptomatic medical student underwent ECG recording for demonstration purposes. What is the abnormality seen in the ECG?

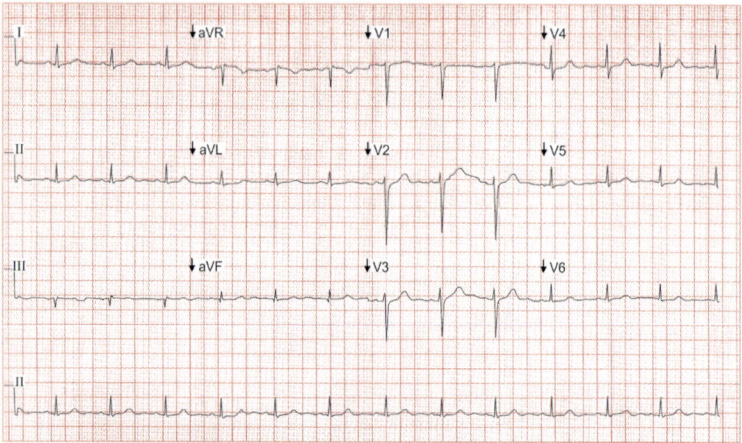

(a) Normal Q waves
(b) Abnormal Q waves
(c) Wide
(d) Low amplitude

Here the ECG shows Q waves in only one lead (lead III). This is within the normal limits, especially given the clinical circumstances.

14. A 56-year-old man presented with chest pain to the emergency. He had sustained myocardial infarction in the past. What does the ECG show?

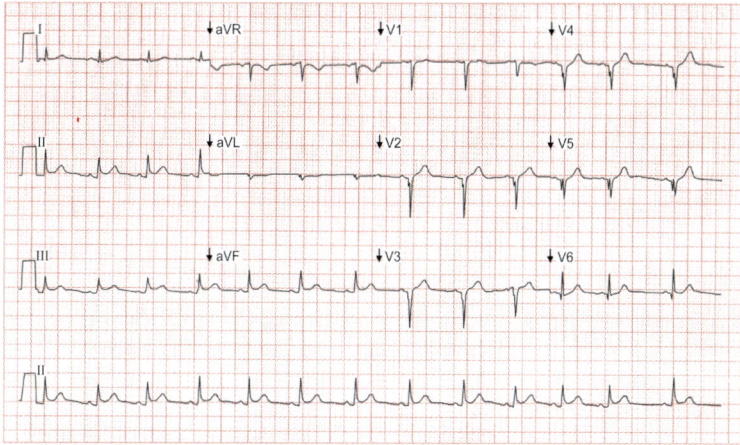

(a) Late progression
(b) Early progression
(c) Normal progression
(d) Artifact

The ECG shows absence of transition by lead V3-V4 and there is predominant R wave only in lead V6. This is an example of late progression of the QRS complex (otherwise called poor progression of the R wave).

15. A 40-year-old man complained of shortness of breath for the past
3 months. He smokes two packs of cigarettes daily for the past
20 years. He is a known patient of hypothyroidism on thyroid
replacement therapy. What does the ECG show?

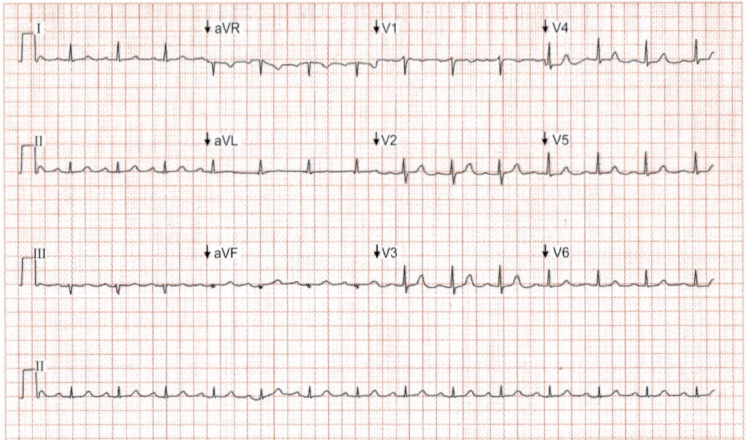

(a) Low amplitude QRS
(b) Tall P waves
(c) Sinus bradycardia
(d) Normal QRS

In the ECG, most of the leads show QRS complexes of
amplitude less than 5 mm in the limb leads and less than
10 mm in the chest leads. This is an example of low-voltage QRS
complexes.

5   T and U Waves

▨ T WAVE

The T waves in the ECG represent repolarization or inactivation of the ventricles. Repolarization process is opposite of depolarization, but is inhomogeneous and slow compared to depolarization. This explains why the T waves are broader and of lesser amplitude than the QRS. If repolarization had been just the opposite of depolarization, the T waves would have been similar to QRS. In addition, the direction of repolarization is opposite to that of depolarization. That is why the T waves are upright instead of being inverted.

Normally, the T wave is smooth and rounded. It has asymmetrical limbs and a blunt apex. The direction of the T wave follows the direction of the QRS complex. So, a predominantly positive QRS complex will have positive T wave and a predominantly negative QRS will have a negative T wave. The T wave is inverted in leads V1–V3 during infancy and, sometimes, this pattern can persist in adulthood also. Like the QRS complex, the amplitude of the T waves also varies widely. The amplitude depends on age, sex and build of the subject. The amplitude of the T waves is usually less than 0.5 mV in the limb leads and less than 1.0 mV in the chest leads. The duration of the T wave is included in the measurement of the QT interval and will be discussed subsequently.

▨ U WAVE

The U wave is seen in the ECG after the T wave as a small rounded wave. It is most prominent in the mid-precordial (chest) leads. The exact genesis of the U wave is not clear. It is thought to represent late repolarization of Purkinje fibers and prolonged repolarization of mid-myocardial cells. The amplitude of the U wave is normally less than that of the T wave and it follows the direction of the T wave. Absence of the U wave is not abnormal.

1. An ECG was recorded in a 35-year-old woman as part of evaluation for an episode of giddiness. What is the finding regarding the T wave?

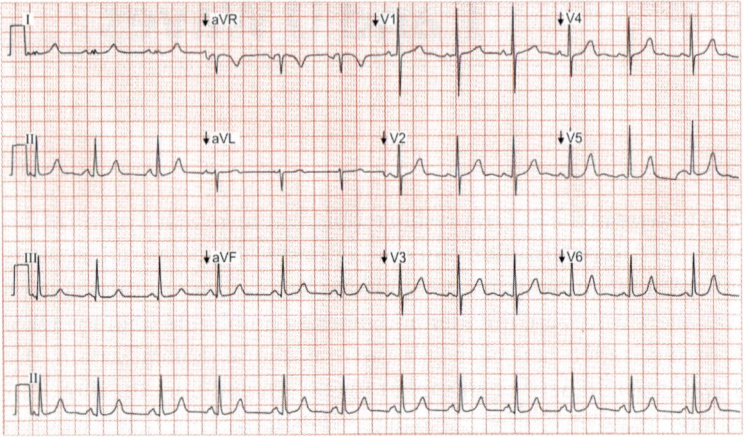

(a) Normal
(b) Tall
(c) Inverted
(d) Broad

The T waves are normal in this ECG. They follow the direction of the QRS complex and the amplitudes are normal.

2. A 50-year-old diabetic woman complained of retrosternal chest discomfort spreading to the left arm and shoulder. What is the abnormality of the T wave seen in the ECG?

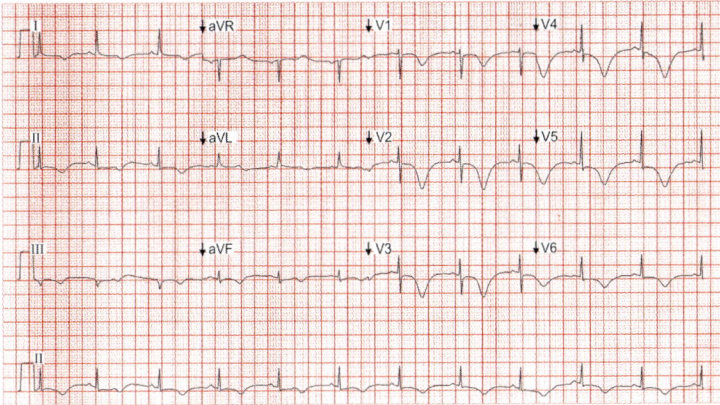

(a) Normal
(b) Tall
(c) Inverted
(d) Notched

In this ECG, the T waves are inverted in all the leads except lead aVR. T wave changes in the ECG are the most nonspecific changes and they have to be always taken in the context of the clinical history and presentation of the patient. The most important cause of T wave inversion is myocardial ischemia and has to be excluded in all such cases. Other causes of T wave inversion include anemia, fever, electrolyte imbalances, drugs, subarachnoid hemorrhage, myocarditis, pulmonary embolism, pericarditis, cardiomyopathy, myocardial infiltrations and hypertrophy, etc. So, the diagnosis of T wave inversion is always correlated with the clinical picture.

3. A 68-year-old man was seen in the emergency for acute onset
    of breathlessness and decreased urine output. He has chronic
    kidney disease and hypertension. His medications include
    enalapril and spironolactone. What is the abnormality of the
    T wave seen in the ECG?

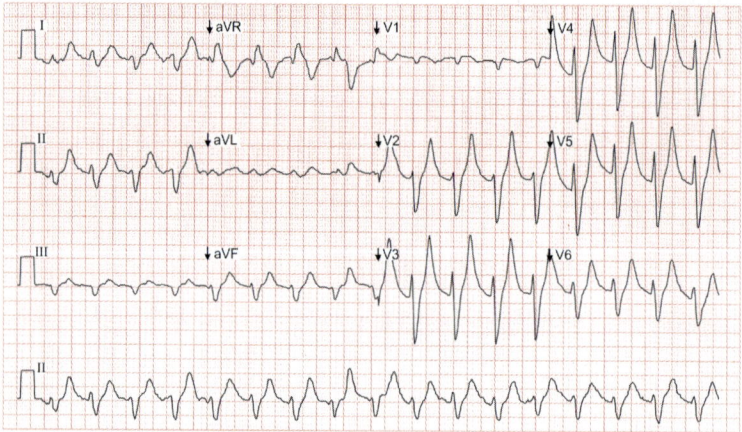

(a) Tall
(b) Inverted
(c) Notched
(d) Broad

The ECG shows tall T waves, especially in the precordial
leads. They are more than 10 mm in amplitude. Tall T waves are
seen in hyperkalemia and hyperacute myocardial infarction.

4. A 57-year-old man diagnosed with dilated cardiomyopathy was started on furosemide for worsening dyspnea. In the follow-up visit, an ECG was recorded. What is the abnormality noticed in the T wave?

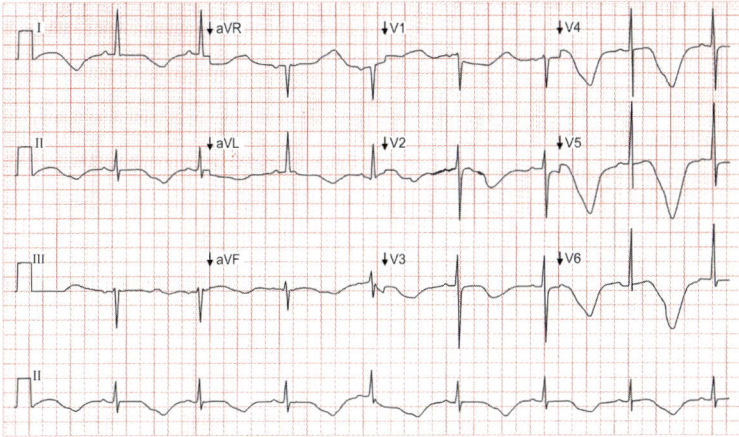

(a) Tall
(b) Normal
(c) Notched
(d) Broad

The T waves in this ECG tracing are broad and inverted. Such broad and inverted T waves are mostly seen in hypokalemia, long QT syndromes and intracranial hemorrhage. Given the clinical setting, one should suspect hypokalemia as the cause of such changes in the ECG.

5. A 50-year-old man was seen in the medicine outpatient department for hypertension. His medications include telmisartan and hydrochlorothiazide. An ECG was done as part of routine evaluation. What is the wave seen after the T wave?

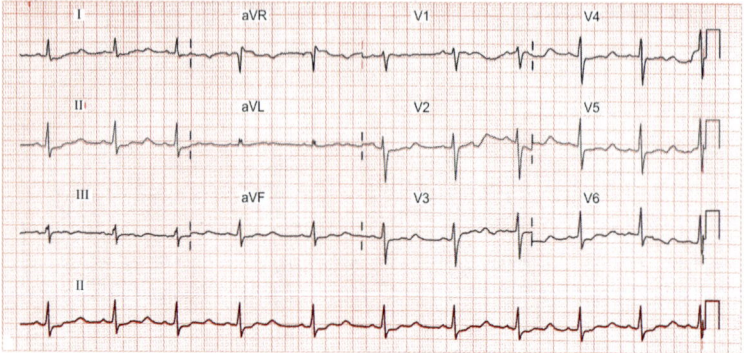

(a) P wave
(b) U wave
(c) Notched T wave
(d) Artifact

This ECG shows a prominent U wave, which is seen as a rounded wave after the T wave. Normally, the U wave is smaller than the T wave or absent. In the tracing, the amplitude of the U waves is larger than that of the T waves. In the clinical scenario given, one should suspect hypokalemia as the patient is on a diuretic.

Chapter

6 ST and PR Segments

ST SEGMENT

The ST segment in the ECG represents the part from the end of the QRS complex to the beginning of the T wave. It is horizontal in the initial part and gradually ascends towards, and merges with, the ascending limb of the T wave. It represents the time during which the ventricles are in the depolarized state and repolarization has just started.

Deviations (elevation or depression) in the ST segment can be normal or abnormal. Elevation by more than 1 mm in two adjacent (anatomically contiguous, leads II and III for example) limb leads or more than 2 mm in two adjacent chest leads is considered significant. Elevation can be with a convexity or concavity upwards. Depression by more than 1 mm in two anatomically contiguous leads is considered significant. Depression can be horizontal, downsloping or upsloping. The deviation of the ST segment from baseline is usually measured at 60 or 80 ms after the J point (junction of QRS complex and the ST segment). The reference baseline is usually the TP segment (portion of ECG between the T wave and the P wave). If the TP segment is not clear, the PR segment (portion of ECG between the P wave and the QRS complex) can be used as the reference baseline.

PR SEGMENT

The PR segment is the part of the ECG between the end of P wave and starting of the QRS complex. It presents the period when the cardiac depolarization wave is travelling across the AV node and the His-Purkinje system. During this time, atrial repolarization is also occurring. However, because of the very small magnitude of atrial repolarization, it is usually not seen as a distinct deflection. The atrial repolarization is masked in the PR segment and the QRS complex.

1. A 50-year-old woman complained of epigastric and retrosternal burning chest pain. She is a diabetic and hypertensive. An ECG was recorded. What is the finding in the ST segment?

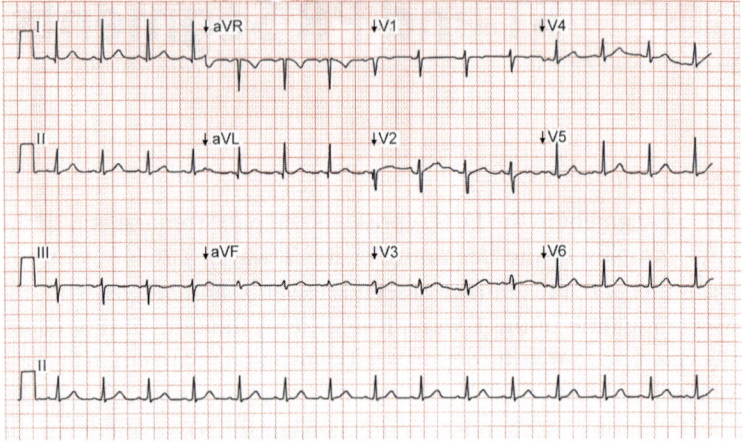

(a) Normal
(b) Elevation
(c) Horizontal depression
(d) Downsloping depression

The ECG tracing shows a normal ST segment. There is neither depression nor elevation of the ST segment. The ST segment gradually merges with the ascending limb of the T wave. Like T wave changes, ST segment changes are also nonspecific and need to be interpreted in the context of the clinical setting.

2. A 46-year-old man complained of severe retrosternal chest discomfort of 30 minutes' duration. What is the finding in the ST segment?

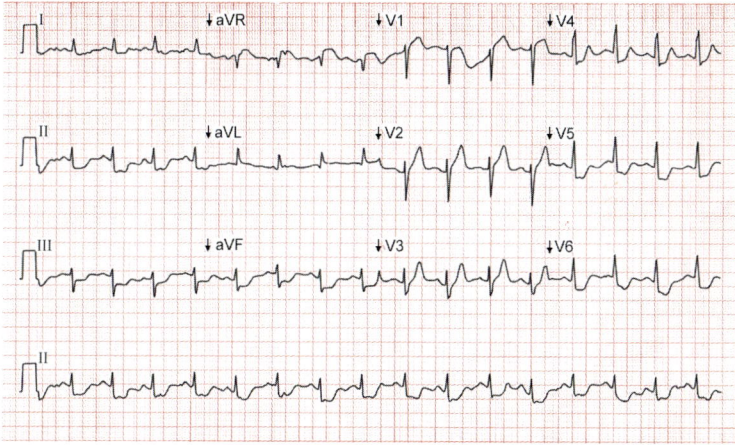

(a) Normal
(b) Elevation
(c) Horizontal depression
(d) Downsloping depression

There is almost 4–5 mm horizontal depression of the ST segment in the inferior and lateral leads. This type of ST depression in association with the clinical symptoms is very suggestive of myocardial ischemia and non-ST elevation myocardial infarction, if the cardiac enzymes are raised. Myocardial ischemia has to be considered in all the cases of horizontal ST depression and chest pain. However, such finding can also occur with myocardial infiltration, hypertrophy and myocarditis.

3. A 66-year-old lady was admitted in the ICU for sudden onset of chest pain and sweating. What is the finding in the ST segment?

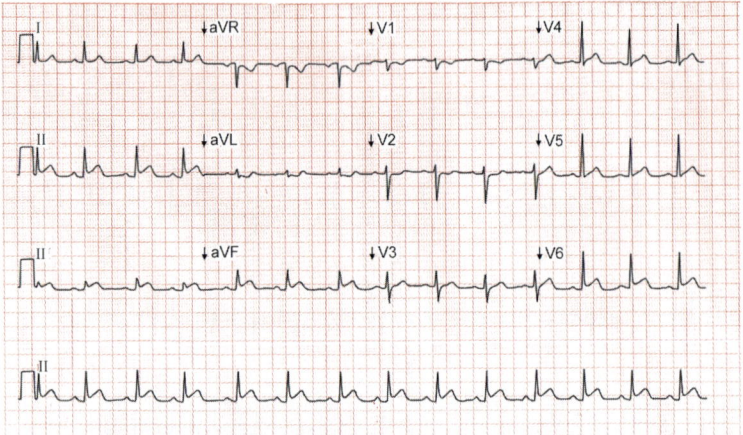

(a) Elevation
(b) Upsloping depression
(c) Horizontal depression
(d) Downsloping depression

The tracing shows ST elevation in leads II, III, aVF and V4–V6. ST elevation in leads V4 and V5 are very subtle but definite. One has to train the eye to pick these subtle ST changes and avoid missing acute myocardial infarction. The ECG changes and clinical picture are suggestive of acute ST elevation myocardial infarction in the inferolateral territory of the left ventricle. ST elevation can also be seen in pericarditis, LV aneurysm and during Prinzmetal angina (vasospastic angina).

4. A 62-year-old man was evaluated for recently detected hypertension. What is the finding in the ST segment?

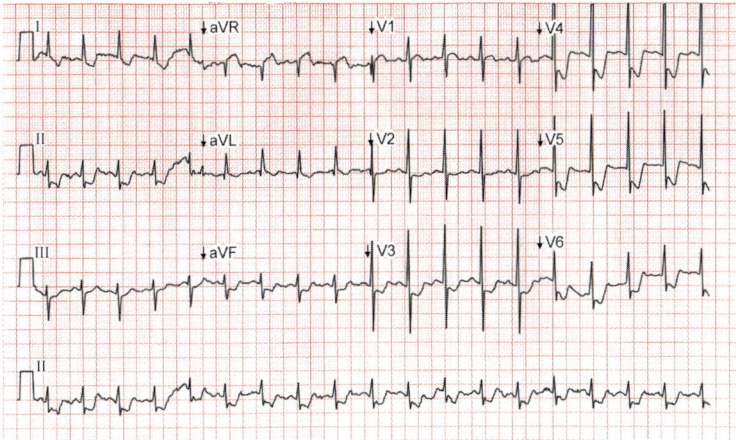

(a) Elevation
(b) Upsloping depression
(c) Horizontal depression
(d) Downsloping depression

The ECG shows ST depression in inferolateral leads. Unlike the previous example, the ST segment depression is downsloping. This again can occur with myocardial ischemia, LV hypertrophy, infiltration and cardiomyopathies. As emphasized earlier, the history of the patient is important in deciding the possible etiology and, in appropriate circumstances, acute myocardial ischemia has to be ruled out.

5. A 35-year-old man underwent ECG for the evaluation of chest pain. What is the abnormality in the ECG?

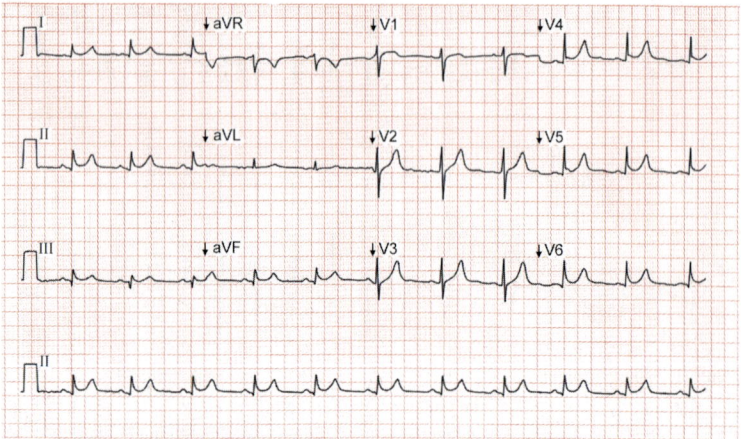

(a) ST elevation
(b) Downsloping ST depression
(c) Upsloping ST depression
(d) Horizontal ST depression

The ECG shows ST elevation in inferolateral leads. The ST segment shows concavity upwards. This is seen with pericarditis and early repolarization syndrome. In acute ST elevation myocardial infarction, the ST segment shows upward convexity. Again, clinical picture has to be taken into account because ST-T changes are nonspecific.

7 PR and QT Intervals

▩ PR INTERVAL

The PR interval is measured from the P wave onset to the onset of the QRS complex. It represents the time taken for the cardiac depolarization to travel through the atria, AV node and the His-Purkinje system. The time taken to traverse the AV node constitutes most of the PR interval because the AV node has a slower conduction velocity. The normal PR interval is 120–200 ms (3 to 5 large squares). PR interval of less than 120 ms is called short PR interval and more than 200 ms is called long PR interval.

▩ QT INTERVAL

The QT interval is measured from the onset of the QRS complex to the end of the T wave. It represents the time taken for ventricular depolarization (activation) and repolarization (inactivation). QT interval varies with the heart rate. The repolarization process shortens with tachycardia and lengthens with bradycardia. Thus, while measuring QT interval, one has to correct (normalize) it for heart rate. There are many formulae available for calculating the corrected QT interval (QTc). The most commonly used formula is the Bazett's formula. According to this formula, QTc is derived by dividing the QT interval by the square root of the RR interval (in seconds). The upper limit of normal QTc interval is 450 ms and it is slightly longer in females. The QT interval is composed of QRS complex, ST segment and the T wave. Prolongation in any of the three components will result in prolonged QT interval. Most commonly, in QT prolongation, T wave duration is prolonged.

1. A 40-year-old asymptomatic man underwent ECG recording as part of preoperative evaluation. What is the finding in the PR interval?

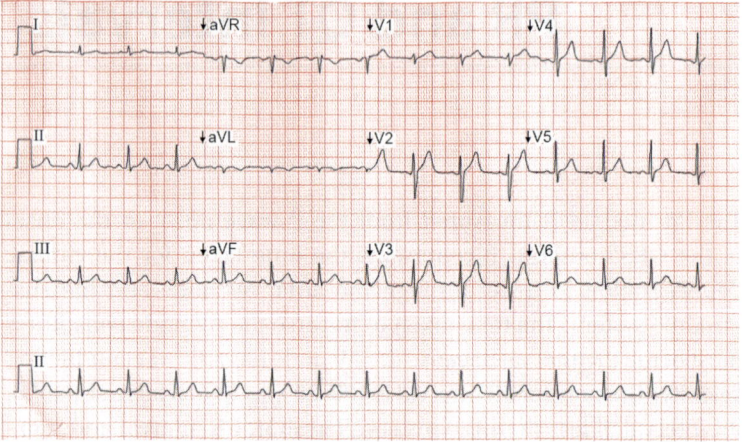

(a) Normal
(b) Prolonged
(c) Short
(d) Cannot be measured

This ECG tracing shows a normal PR interval. The PR interval is 160 ms (there are 4 small squares from the onset of P wave to the onset of the QRS complex).

2. A 55-year-old man complained of tiredness and weakness. He is on treatment for hypertension and his dose of metoprolol was increased during the last visit. What is the finding in the PR interval?

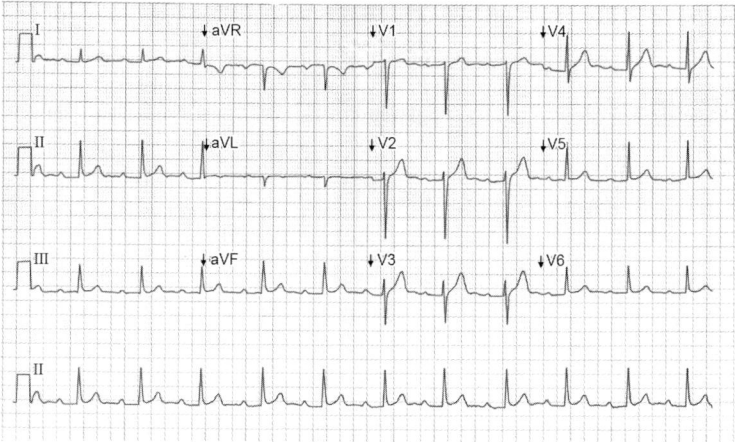

(a) Short
(b) Prolonged and constant
(c) Prolonged and varying
(d) Cannot be measured reliably

The PR interval in this ECG is prolonged and measures 320 ms. The PR interval is constant throughout the tracing. This is a case of abnormal PR interval. The normal PR interval measures between 120 and 200 ms. It is best to look at the PR interval in the rhythm strip to determine any variations in the interval. PR interval prolongation occurs when there is delay in the conduction of impulses from the atria to the ventricle. The delay can be in the atrium, AV node or the infranodal tissues.

3. A 34-year-old athlete was noticed to have irregular pulse during routine examination and an ECG was recorded. What is the finding regarding PR interval?

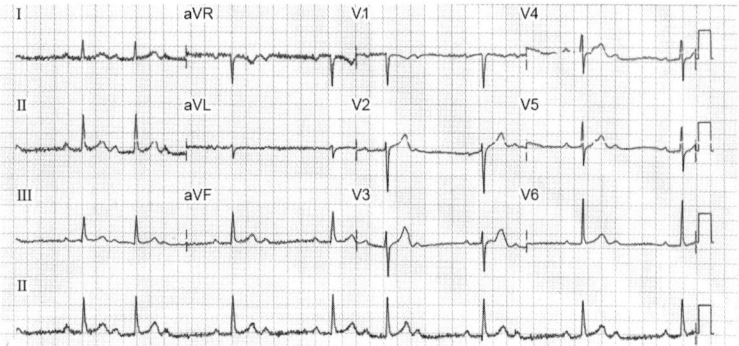

(a) Normal
(b) Prolonged and constant
(c) Prolonged and varying
(d) Cannot be measured reliably

This tracing shows again prolonged PR interval (>200 ms) and also the PR interval keeps varying. At times, the P wave is not followed by QRS complex and the PR interval cannot be measured. The variation in the PR interval gives rise to the irregularity in the rhythm. The prolonged and varying PR interval is caused by delay and intermittent block in the conduction from atria to the ventricles. We will discuss in detail about this in later sections.

4. A 70-year-old man was seen in the emergency department for recurrent episodes of giddiness and syncope. What is the finding regarding PR interval in the ECG?

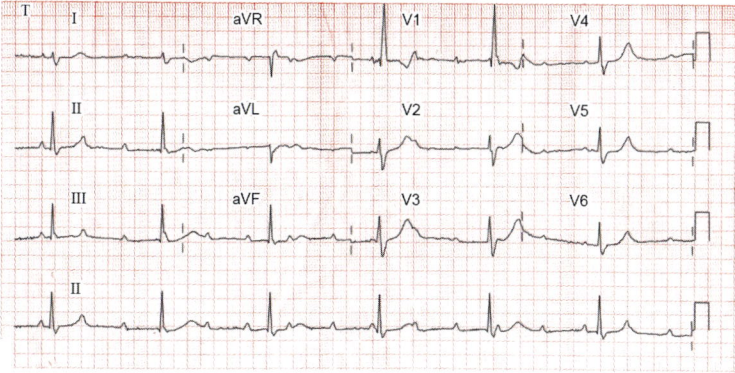

(a) Normal
(b) Prolonged and constant
(c) Prolonged and varying
(d) Cannot be measured reliably

In this ECG, one cannot reliably measure the PR interval as there is no relation between the P wave and the QRS complex. P wave is seen marching through the QRS complexes. In other words, the P waves are not conducted to the ventricles. The ventricles have their own rhythm and the atria their own. Ventricular rate (calculated from R to R interval) is approximately 38 beats per minute and the atrial rate (calculated from P to P interval) is 100 beats per minute.

5. A 32-year-old lady complained of recurrent episodes of palpitations associated with sweating and giddiness. A resting 12 lead ECG was recorded. What is the finding regarding PR interval in the ECG?

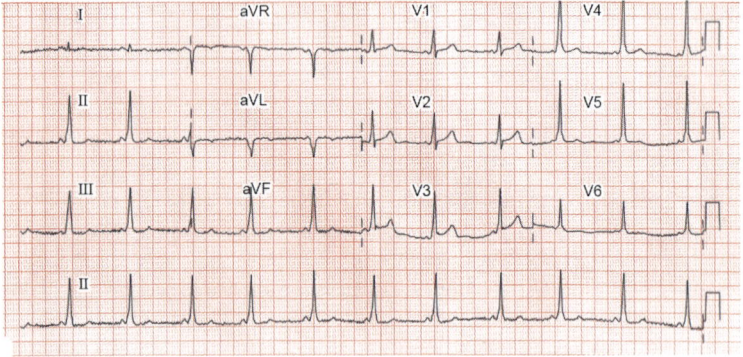

(a) Normal
(b) Short
(c) Prolonged
(d) Cannot be measured reliably

In this ECG, the PR interval is short (less than 120 ms). Each P wave is consistently followed by a QRS complex after a constant, though short, PR interval. This indicates that either the conduction through the AV node is enhanced or there is an alternate fast-conducting route to the ventricles. Sometimes an accelerated junctional rhythm with isorhythmic AV dissociation can also have such apparent short PR interval. In the present case, the QRS complex is also wide with an initial slurring. This is suggestive of an accessory pathway present between the atria and the ventricles. In case of accelerated junctional rhythm with apparent short PR interval, the QRS will be narrow.

6. A 50-year-old man was seen in the medicine outpatient department for hypertension. His medications include telmisartan and hydrochlorothiazide. An ECG was done as part of routine evaluation. What is the finding regarding the QT interval in the ECG?

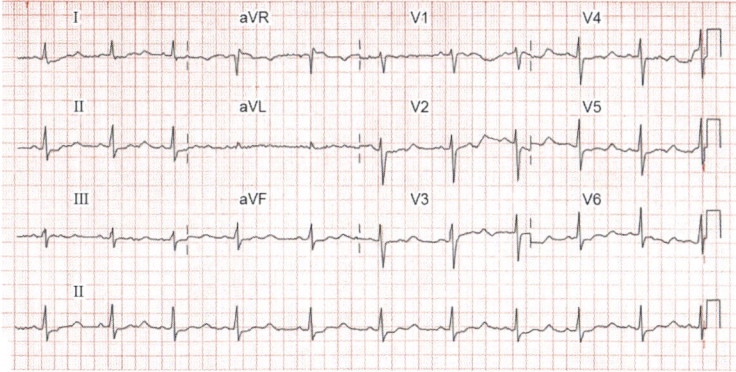

(a) Cannot be measured
(b) Shortened
(c) Normal
(d) Absent

In this ECG, the end of T wave cannot be seen reliably because there is a prominent U wave. In the calculation of the QT interval, U waves are not included. One of the methods to measure the QT interval is to draw a tangent from the downslope of the T wave and determine the intersection point with the baseline. Measuring from the onset of the QRS complex to this intersection point will give the QT interval, which should be corrected for the heart rate. In this tracing, prominent U waves are abnormal and hypokalemia is probable in the given clinical setting. The QT interval is normal.

7. A 57-year-old man diagnosed with dilated cardiomyopathy was started on furosemide for worsening dyspnea. In the follow-up visit, an ECG was recorded. What is the abnormality noticed in the QT interval?

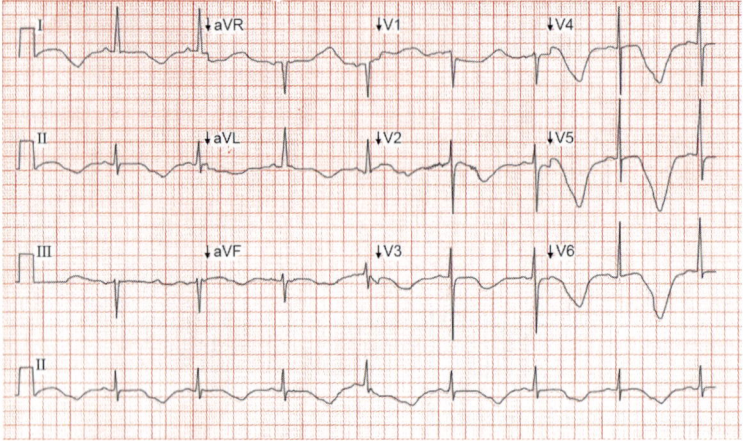

(a) Normal
(b) Prolonged
(c) Shortened
(d) Absent

In this ECG, the QT interval is grossly prolonged. The width of the T wave is markedly increased, contributing to the prolonged QT interval. QT interval can also be prolonged due to increased duration of the ST segment or the QRS complex. Intracranial hemorrhages are an important cause of bizarre T waves and long QT interval. The patient's clinical picture is suggestive of hypokalemia from diuretic use.

8. A 36-year-old woman presented with weakness of all four limbs and inability to walk. She gives history of previous episodes in the past precipitated by high carbohydrate meals. An ECG was recorded which showed a prolonged corrected QT interval. Which component of QT interval is prolonged?

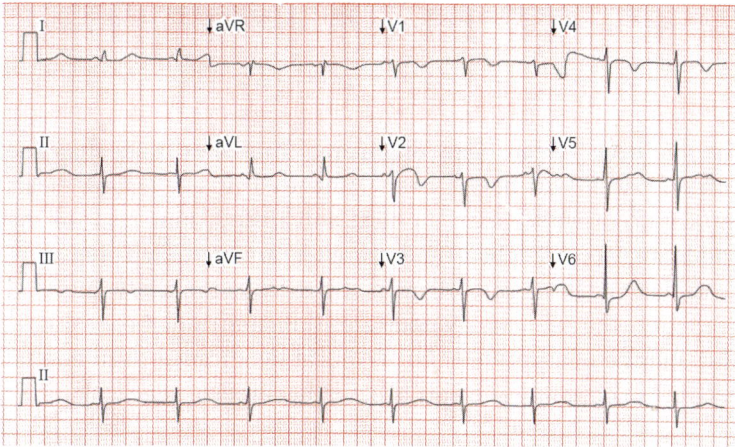

(a) QRS complex
(b) ST segment
(c) T wave
(d) All components

In this ECG, the QT interval is prolonged and the prolongation is caused by increased duration of the T wave. The clinical picture is suggestive of hypokalemia with periodic paralysis. As we discussed earlier, QT prolongation can occur by prolongation of the QRS complex or the ST segment or the T wave or a combination of all these components. Prolongation of the QRS occurs with class IC antiarrhythmic drugs. Prolongation of the ST segment is seen with hypocalcemia. Prolongation of the T waves occurs with hypokalemia, intracranial hemorrhage etc.

8 Ectopic Beats, Escape Beats and Rhythms

▨ ECTOPIC (PREMATURE) BEATS

'Ectopic beats' mean beats originating from sites other than the normal pacemaker of the heart (sinoatrial node). Ectopic beats usually occur earlier than the next anticipated sinus beat (or the dominant pacemaker beat) and, therefore, are also called premature beats. Ectopic beats can originate anywhere in the heart. They can come from the atria, the AV node area (junction) and the ventricles. They may be nonspecific or be of clinical significance. Even normal people can have some ectopic beats, either atrial or ventricular.

Supraventricular Ectopic Beats

Atrial and junctional ectopic beats (supraventricular) are identified by narrow QRS complex (normal QRS duration) beats that occur early. Since impulses originating from above the level of bundle of His will conduct to ventricles through the normal conduction system, atrial and junctional beats will result in a normal QRS complex. Atrial ectopic beats are recognized by the presence of abnormal P waves preceding the QRS complex. Sometimes, the P wave will be on top of the previous T wave and is identified by the appearance of a 'peaked' T wave (P on T).

Failure to identify a definite P wave preceding the QRS complex makes the ectopic beat of junctional origin. Presence of inverted P waves in leads II, III and aVF immediately after the QRS also is suggestive of junctional ectopic beat. In the presence of inverted P waves preceding the QRS, a very short PR interval is suggestive of a junctional beat. The P waves are inverted in case of junctional beats because an impulse originating from the junctional area will conduct to the atria retrogradely from inferior to superior direction (reverse of normal). This will result in inverted P waves. Thus, the junctional beats are identified by a narrow QRS complex and the presence of inverted P following the QRS, inverted P wave with a short PR interval preceding the QRS or the absence of P waves for the corresponding QRS complex.

Ventricular Ectopic Beats

Ventricular ectopic beats are identified by the presence of wide QRS without preceding P waves. If P waves are present, they are not related to the QRS (PR interval will be abnormal). Ventricular ectopic beat can originate from any part of the ventricle and then spread from there to activate the rest of the ventricles. In this instance, the conduction is not occurring through the normal conduction system. It is occurring by way of muscle-to-muscle conduction, which is slow compared to conduction through the His-Purkinje system. This is the reason why beats originating from the ventricles result in wide and notched QRS complexes.

Supraventricular ectopic beats are followed by a non-compensatory pause. This means that the time interval between the normal-to-normal beat encompassing the ectopic beat is less than twice the RR interval (interval between two consecutive normal beats). On the other hand, the ventricular ectopic beats are followed by fully compensated pauses. Here the time interval between the normal-to-normal beat encompassing the ectopic beat is twice the normal RR interval.

▓ WIDE QRS COMPLEX BEATS

Ventricular beats manifest as wide QRS complexes in the ECG. However, all wide beats are not of ventricular origin. We will discuss here about the wide complex beat, though they do not strictly fall under the category of ectopic beats. Supraventricular beats can be wide whenever ventricular conduction of the impulse is abnormal. This happens when there is an abnormal conduction pathway between the atria and ventricle (accessory pathway) or when there is impaired conduction in the bundle branches (physiologic or pathologic). Another cause of wide complex are artificial ventricular paced beats.

Pre-excited Beats

When there is an extra conduction pathway (accessory pathway) between the atria and ventricles, the ventricles will be activated by both the AV node and the accessory pathway. The accessory pathway inserts into the ventricular myocardium and conduction along it will result in activation of the myocardium directly. The activation then spreads from there to the rest of the myocardium, resulting in abnormal activation of the ventricles. This results in an abnormal wide QRS complex. The degree of widening will depend on the amount of myocardium activated by the accessory pathway. The more the amount of myocardial activation through the accessory pathway, the wider the QRS complex will be. This can be differentiated from the ventricular ectopic by the presence of preceding P wave, short PR interval and delta wave (slurred initial component of the QRS representing ventricular activation by way of the accessory pathway).

Bundle Branch Block

The QRS complexes will also be wide when there is conduction abnormality of the bundle branches. When conduction in one of the bundles is impaired or absent, activation of the ventricles occurs by the contralateral bundle. This results in normal activation of the contralateral ventricle. However, activation of the ipsilateral ventricle occurs from the contralateral ventricle by way of muscle-to-muscle conduction. This leads to a wide QRS complex. Conduction abnormality in the bundles may be physiologic and transient or pathologic and fixed. Pathologic conduction defect occurs when there is disease and fibrosis of the bundle branches. Physiologic conduction defect (aberrant conduction) occurs at faster rates and resolves once the rate normalizes. An ectopic beat may be conducted with aberrancy because it encroaches on the refractory period of one of the bundles. The early beat (ectopic) arrives at the bundle of His when the bundle branches have not fully recovered from the previous depolarization. This results in conduction of the impulse along the bundle which has recovered and block in the bundle which has not recovered fully. Again this will lead to abnormal activation of the ventricles leading to a wide QRS complex. In case of bundle branch block, the initial activation is normal (contralateral to the bundle branch block) and the terminal activation is abnormal (ipsilateral to the bundle branch block). This will result in sharp deflections of the initial portion of QRS and slurred deflections of the terminal portion of the QRS complex. Also since only the right or left bundle is involved, there can be only two specific patterns of QRS resulting from the bundle branch block (bundle branch block morphology will be discussed later). So, differentiation from ventricular ectopic is by way of recognizing the specific morphology with initial rapid ventricular activation (initial sharp inscription of the QRS) and the presence of preceding P wave with normal or prolonged PR interval.

Ventricular Paced Beat

Ventricular paced beat will have wide complex. The ventricle is stimulated at a particular site and the impulse travels from there to activate the rest of the ventricle. Since the impulse conducts through the ventricular cells, the conduction is prolonged and so the QRS is wide. Ventricular paced beat is identified by the presence of pacing stimulus preceding the QRS complex.

ESCAPE BEATS AND RHYTHMS

Escape beat occurs whenever there is failure of the primary driving rhythm, which is normally the SA node. When there is slowing of the sinus node, either due to physiological or pathological causes, subsidiary pacemakers tend to take control of the heart rhythm. So, escape beats occur later than the anticipated normal beat, unlike ectopic beats that occur earlier. Also in escape beat, the pause in the rhythm occurs before the beat while in ectopic beats, the pause occurs after the beat.

As discussed earlier, the rate of firing of the SA node is higher than any focus in rest of the conduction system. So, under normal conditions, the SA node is the pacemaker of the heart. The normal rate of depolarization of the SA node is 60 to 100 per minute. The rate of firing of the AV junction area is 40 to 60 per minute and the Purkinje fibers in the ventricles depolarize at rates less than 40 per minute. When the rate of the SA node falls to less than 60 per minute, the AV junction takes over and if that also fails, then the ventricles take over. Junctional rhythms are quite stable and reliable. Ventricular rhythm is unstable and unreliable.

Junctional rate of more than 60 per minute but less than 100 per minute is called accelerated junctional rhythm. A junctional rate more than 100 beats per minute is called junctional tachycardia. A ventricular rate between 40 and 100 per minute is called accelerated ventricular rhythm and a rate more than 100 per minute is called ventricular tachycardia.

1. A 35-year-old man complained of episodes of palpitations and instances of skipped heart beats. What does the 12 lead ECG show?

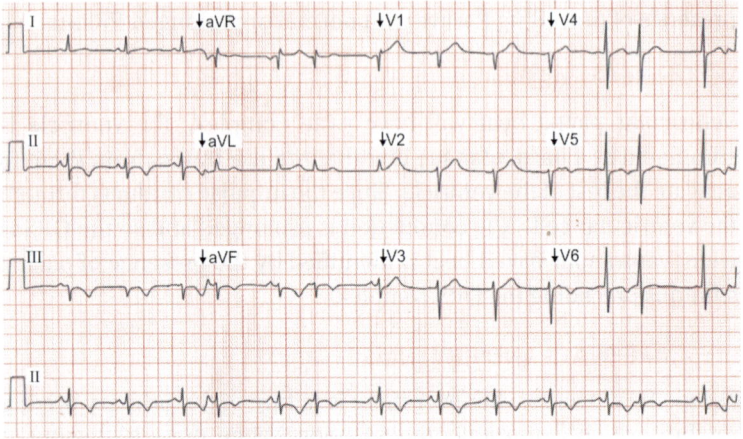

(a) Atrial ectopic beat
(b) Ventricular ectopic beat
(c) Junctional ectopic beat
(d) Ventricular escape beat

Ectopic beats are better observed in the rhythm strip. In the ECG, there are three ectopic beats (beat numbers 4, 6, and 12 in the rhythm strip at the bottom) and these are followed by a pause. The QRS complexes of these beats are narrow and similar to the normal beats. The pause following the ectopic beats is noncompensatory, i.e. the RR interval encompassing the ectopic beat is less than twice the normal RR interval (interval between two consecutive normally occurring beats). These features are suggestive of supraventricular ectopic. The second ectopic (sixth beat in the rhythm strip) is preceded by a P wave that falls on the T wave, making the T wave more negative and peaked as compared to other T waves. Thus, the ectopic beat is an atrial ectopic beat. Atrial ectopic beats can be seen in normal individuals, but are more frequent in those with diseased atria.

2. A 56-year-old man complained of pricking chest pain and episodes of fluttering in the chest. What does the 12 lead ECG show?

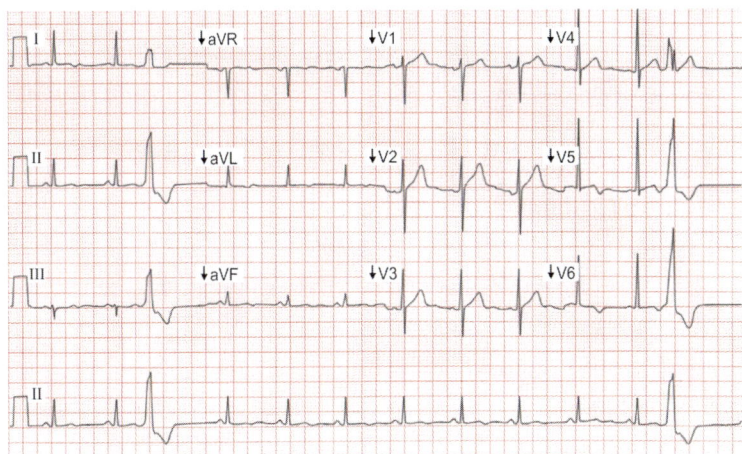

(a) Atrial ectopic beat
(b) Ventricular ectopic beat
(c) Junctional ectopic beat
(d) Atrial escape beat

The rhythm strip shows two early occurring beats followed by a pause. This is suggestive of an ectopic beat. The ectopic beat shows wide QRS complex and is not preceded by any P waves. Also the pause following the beat is fully compensated, i.e. the RR interval encompassing the ectopic beat is twice the normal RR interval. These features are suggestive of ventricular ectopic beat. A few ventricular ectopic beats can be seen in normal individuals. However, frequent ventricular ectopics are abnormal and need further evaluation.

3. A 70-year-old woman was admitted in the ICU for congestive cardiac failure. She is a known patient of dilated cardiomyopathy. The monitor showed irregular QRS complexes and an ECG was recorded. What does the ECG show?

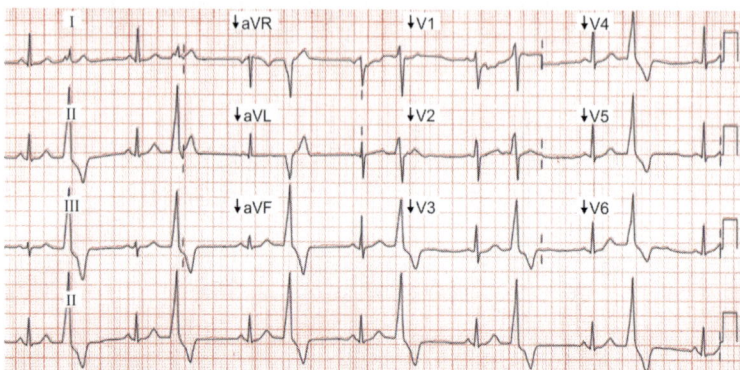

(a) Ventricular bigeminy
(b) Ventricular trigeminy
(c) Ventricular couplets
(d) Nonsustained ventricular tachycardia

The rhythm strip shows frequent ectopic beats. The beats are wide and are not preceded by any P waves. This is suggestive of ventricular ectopic beats. In this example, the ventricular ectopic beats are alternating with normal beats. This pattern is called ventricular bigeminy. This will result in pulsus bigeminy clinically or sometimes if the contractions due to ventricular ectopics are weak, it may not result in a frequent pulse and can be mistaken for bradycardia. If the ventricular ectopic beats occur regularly after every second normal beat, then the pattern is called trigeminy.

4. A 25-year-old female complained of recurrent episodes of palpitations and an episode of syncope. She was noticed to have irregular pulse by her physician and was referred for cardiac evaluation. What does the ECG show?

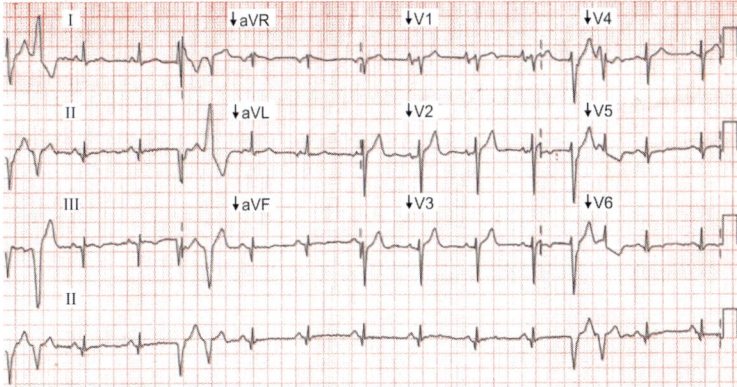

(a) Ventricular bigemeny
(b) Atrial bigeminy
(c) Ventricular couplet
(d) Atrial couplet

The rhythm strip shows frequent ectopic beats. The beats are wide and are not preceded by any P waves. This is suggestive of ventricular ectopic beats. In this example, the ventricular ectopic beats are occurring in pairs. This pattern is called ventricular couplets. If there are consecutive three ventricular ectopics, then it is called triplet. If there are more than three in a row, it qualifies for ventricular tachycardia. In the absence of heart disease and symptoms, most of the isolated ectopics do not need any specific treatment.

5. A 75-year-old man complained of recurrent episodes of giddiness and presyncope. An ECG was done as part of evaluation. What does the ECG show?

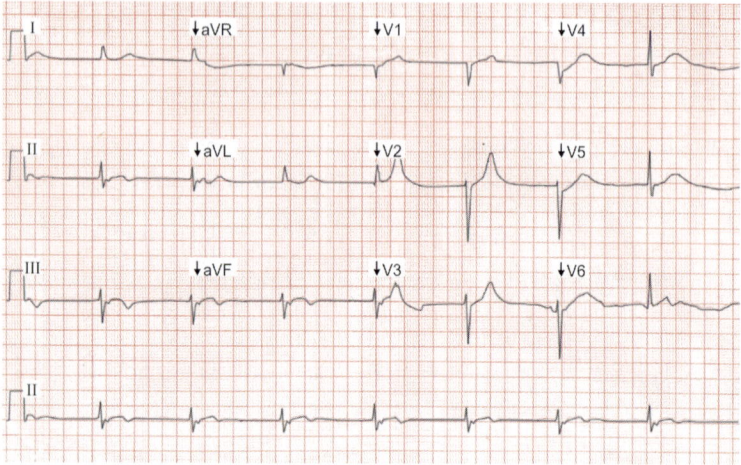

(a) Atrial escape beat
(b) Ventricular escape beat
(c) Junctional escape beat
(d) Idioventricular rhythm

The ECG shows QRS complexes occurring at a regular interval at the rate of approximately 45 beats per minute, best seen in the rhythm strip. QRS complexes are not preceded by any P wave. This is suggestive of junctional rhythm. In case of junctional rhythm, a site in the AV junction area fires and then conducts down to ventricles antegradely and atria retrogradely. Atrial activation can occur just before, during or after the ventricular activation. Since the ventricles are activated by way of the normal conduction system, the activation will be normal and so the QRS complex will be normal. Since the atria are activated from inferior to superior direction, the P waves will be inverted in inferior leads. In the ECG shown, there is an inverted P wave just at the end of QRS seen in leads II, III and aVF. Junctional rhythm occurs when there is failure of the sinus node to initiate the rhythm.

6. A 24-year-old male complained of recurrent episodes of palpitations. An ECG was recorded and it showed wide QRS complexes. What is the cause of the wide QRS complex?

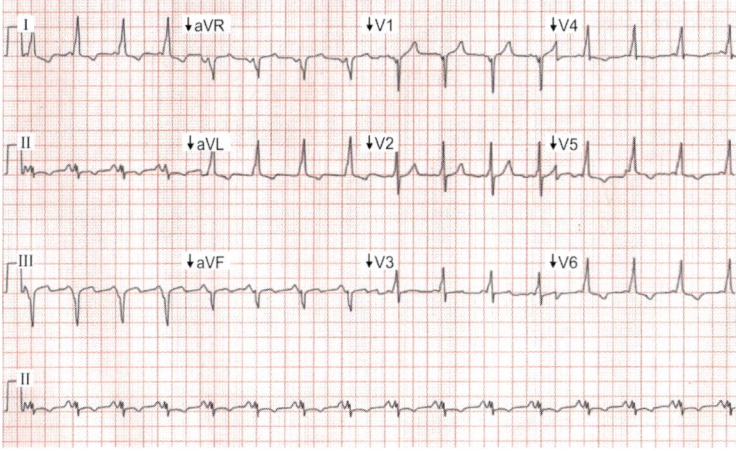

(a) Pre-excitation
(b) Ventricular ectopic
(c) Aberrant conduction
(d) Artifact

The ECG shows regular wide QRS complex preceded by P wave with a short PR interval. The short PR interval and the initial slurring of the QRS (delta wave) are suggestive of pre-excitation. Ventricular pre-excitation occurs when a part of ventricle is activated by an accessory AV conduction tissue before activation by His-Purkinje system. This early activation causes the short PR interval and activation of ventricle by way of the accessory pathway results in delta wave, contributing to the wide QRS complex. Artifact can sometimes be mistaken for wide complex QRS beats if not carefully scrutinized. ECG shown here is a clean recording and there is no evidence of artifact. Aberrant conduction usually will show specific QRS morphology, either RBBB or LBBB, which is not seen in the tracing. Ventricular ectopics will not have a constant relation to the preceding P waves.

7. A 50-year-old man underwent ECG recording for the evaluation of left-sided chest pain. He is a known patient of coronary artery disease and had sustained myocardial infarction in the past. ECG showed a wide complex QRS beat. What is the cause of the wide complex?

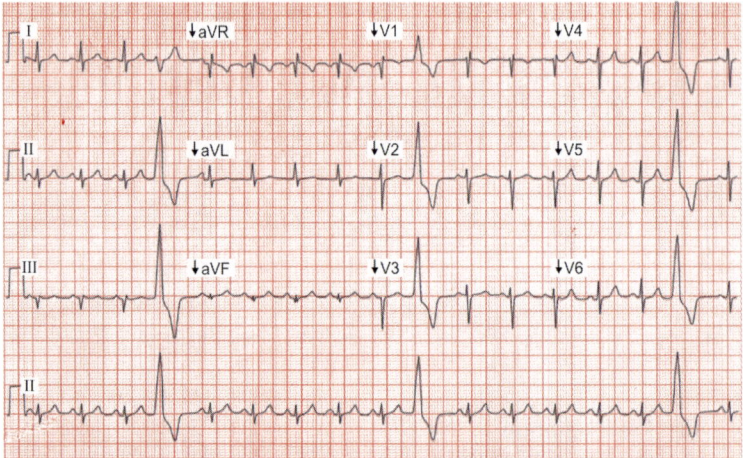

(a) Pre-excitation
(b) Ventricular ectopic beat
(c) Aberrant conduction
(d) Artifact

The ECG shows sinus tachycardia and three wide complex beats. The wide complex beats are not preceded by any P waves and are early in timing. This is suggestive of ventricular ectopic beat. Pre-excited beats will have a preceding P wave, short PR interval and delta waves. Aberrant beats will have specific QRS morphology, either RBBB or LBBB, and will be preceded by P waves. Artifact is unlikely as the tracing is clean. Ventricular paced beats are also wide complex beats but they will be preceding by a pacemaker spike (stimulus artifact).

8. A 40-year-old man underwent ECG recording during preoperative evaluation. The intern noticed that there was a wide complex QRS in the ECG and was concerned about it. What is the genesis of the wide complex QRS beat?

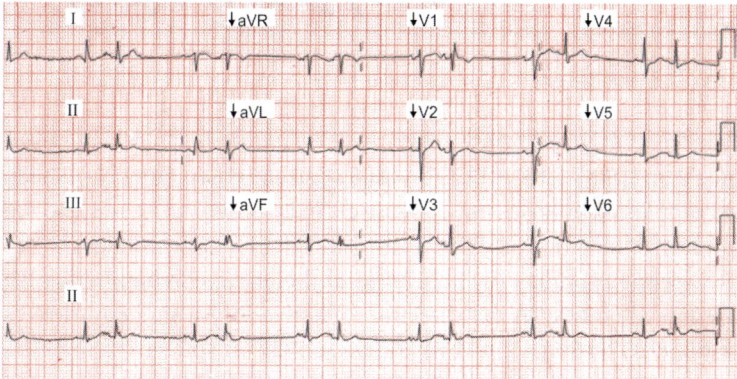

(a) Pre-excitation
(b) Ventricular ectopic beat
(c) Aberrant conduction
(d) Artifact

The ECG shows wide complex beats alternating with narrow complex beats (normal). The wide complex beats are preceded by P waves and normal PR interval. There is no delta wave and the complexes show RBBB pattern (rsR') in lead V1. This is suggestive of aberrant conduction. The P waves occur early and, hence, this is an example of atrial ectopic beats in bigeminy pattern with aberrant conduction. Atrial ectopic beats conduct to the ventricles earlier than normal. At this time, the right bundle is still in refractory period and, hence, the beat conducts down with RBBB pattern. This is physiological and normal.

Chamber Enlargement and Hypertrophy

Enlargement/hypertrophy of the cardiac chambers can be diagnosed based on characteristic ECG findings. Cardiac enlargement is usually accompanied by an increase in muscle mass and so an increase in the amount of electrical activity. This results in increased voltages in the ECG signal produced by activation of the enlarged chambers. Also there is alteration in the direction of activation, which contributes to the ECG findings. However, relying solely on voltages in the ECG is very nonspecific and can lead to wrong conclusions. The recorded voltage is dependent on the build of patient, age of the patient and the amount of intervening lung tissue between the heart and recording electrodes.

ATRIAL ENLARGEMENT

As mentioned earlier, the best leads to look at while evaluating atrial abnormalities are lead II and lead V1. Right atrial enlargement is diagnosed when the P wave amplitude is more than 2.5 mm in lead II and more than 1.5 mm in lead V1. The duration of P wave is not affected by right atrial enlargement as the right atrial activation is represented by initial two-thirds of the P wave and any further increase in duration generally falls within the last one-third of the P wave. Left atrial enlargement will prolong the duration of the P wave. The P wave duration will be increased to more than 2.5 mm (100 ms) in lead II and the terminal (negative) deflection in lead V1 will be more than 1 mm in depth and 0.04 s in duration. Left atrial enlargement will also produce notching of the P wave with two peaks in lead II. Duration of the notch of more than 0.04 seconds is very specific for left atrial enlargement. Biatrial enlargement will show features of both right and left atrial enlargements in the ECG.

▧ VENTRICULAR ENLARGEMENT

Ventricular enlargement is diagnosed based on findings in both the chest and limb leads. As discussed before, there will be an increase in the amount of electrical activity generated by the hypertrophied/enlarged ventricles and it is seen in the ECG as increased amplitudes of the QRS complex. During normal activation of the ventricles, the right ventricular activation is overshadowed by the dominant left ventricular activation. Hence, the right ventricular activation is not obvious on the 12 lead ECG. The normal QRS complex is the result of initial septal activation (left to right direction), activation of both ventricles (dominated by left ventricle and, hence, leftward and posterior direction) and finally the posterobasal ventricles (superior direction). There are several criteria to diagnose ventricular hypertrophy. As a starter, it is best to remember one or two and apply them regularly.

Right ventricular activation is prolonged in case of right ventricular hypertrophy and is seen in right-sided lead as tall R waves and deep S waves in left-sided leads. RVH is diagnosed when the sum of R wave in lead V1 and deepest S wave in lead I or V6 is more than 11 mm (Sokolow-Lyon criteria). R wave more than 7 mm in V1 or R' wave more than 15 mm in the presence of RBBB is also suggestive of RVH.

Left ventricular enlargement is diagnosed if the sum of S wave in lead V1 and R wave in lead V5 or V6 is more than 35 mm or R wave of more than 26 mm in lead V5 or V6 (Sokolow-Lyon criteria). LVH is also suggested by an R wave of more than 11 mm in lead aVL. Biventricular enlargement is diagnosed by presence of criteria for both RVH and LVH.

1. A 23-year-old woman presented with one episode of mild hemoptysis. She gives history of dyspnea on exertion for the past 3 years and was diagnosed to have rheumatic heart disease. An ECG was done during the evaluation. Which is the heart chamber that is likely abnormal?

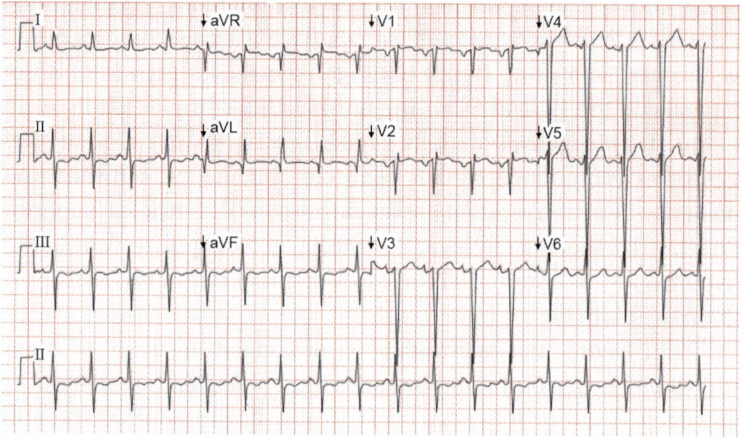

(a) Right atrium
(b) Left atrium
(c) Right and left atria
(d) None

The ECG shows a prominent negative component of the P wave in lead V1. The P wave is more than 1 mm in depth and width in lead V1. This is suggestive of the left atrial enlargement. In lead II, though the duration of the P wave is within normal limits, there is definite notching of the contour, which is supportive of the left atrial enlargement. Patient's history also suggests that she is likely to have left atrial enlargement.

2. A 65-year-old man presented with shortness of breath for the past
    1 year. He smokes 2 packs of cigarette daily for the past 45 years.
    Which chamber of the heart is abnormal based on the recorded
    ECG?

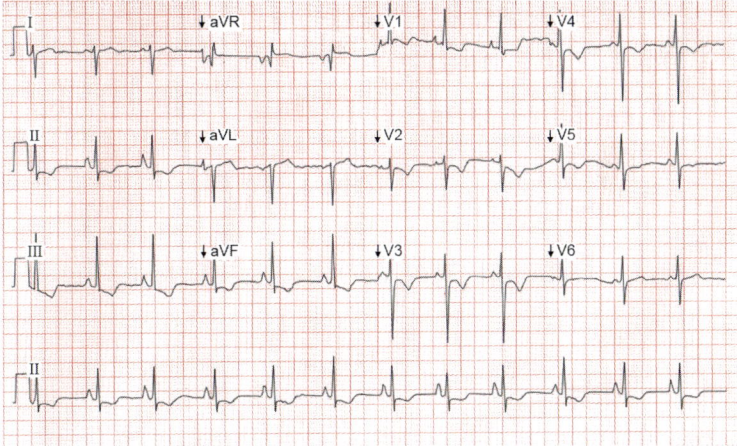

(a) Right atrium
(b) Left atrium
(c) Right and left atria
(d) Left ventricle

The ECG shows tall peaked P waves in leads II, III and aVF.
The height of the P wave in these leads is more than 2.5 mm. In
lead V1, there is a positive P wave with a height of more than
1.5 mm. These features are suggestive of right atrial enlargement.
The patient probably has chronic obstructive airway disease
because of smoking. This has led to pulmonary artery
hypertension and subsequent right atrial enlargement.

3. A 50-year-old man was seen in the cardiac OPD for routine evaluation of his cardiac status. He is a known patient of bicuspid aortic valve with moderate-to-severe aortic stenosis. Which chamber of the heart is likely enlarged based on the ECG?

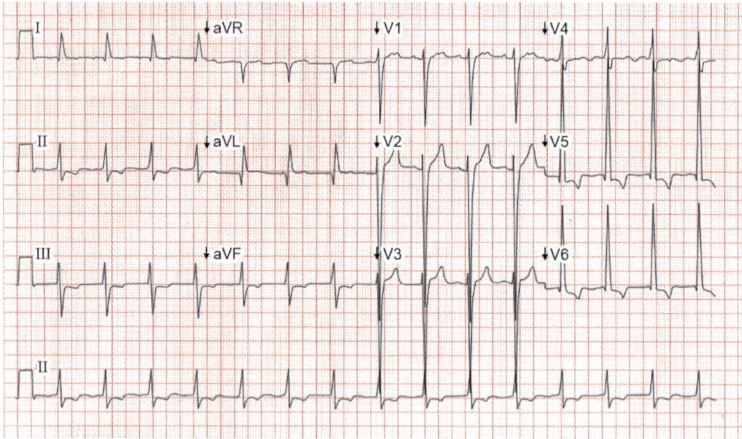

(a) Right atrium
(b) Left atrium
(c) Right ventricle
(d) Left ventricle

The ECG shows tall R waves in leads V5 and V6 with deep S waves in leads V1-V3. The sum of S in lead V1/V2 and R wave in lead V5/V6 is more than 35 mm. This is suggestive of left ventricular hypertrophy. Also the height of R wave in lead V5/V6 is more than 26 mm, again suggestive of left ventricular hypertrophy. The patient has moderate-to-severe aortic stenosis and this can cause left ventricular hypertrophy. The P wave morphology is not suggestive of the right or left atrial enlargement.

4. A 30-year-old woman presented with shortness of breath and swelling of both feet for the past 2 months. Cardiovascular examination revealed a loud pulmonary component of the second heart sound and a short ejection systolic murmur. Which chamber of the heart is likely to be abnormal based on the ECG?

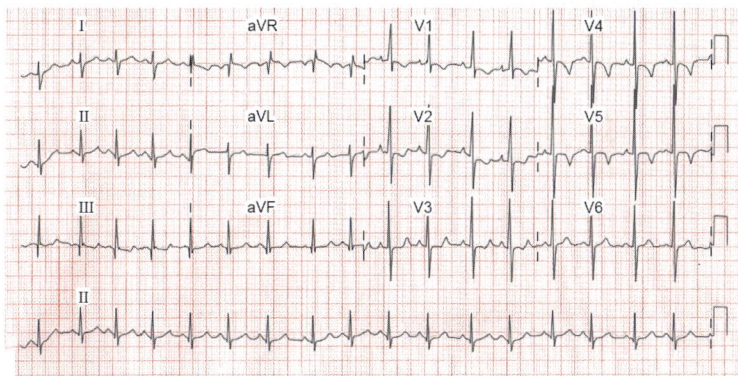

(a) Right atrium
(b) Left atrium
(c) Right ventricle
(d) Left ventricle

The ECG shows tall R wave in lead V1 and prominent S waves in lead I and V6. The amplitude of the R wave in lead V1 is more than 7 mm and the sum of R wave in lead V1 and S wave in lead V6 is more than 11 mm. These features are suggestive of right ventricular enlargement.

Based on the history and clinical features, the patient probably has pulmonary hypertension, which has caused the right ventricular enlargement.

5. A 23-year-old woman was detected to have a mid-diastolic murmur at the apex with loud first heart sound and pansystolic murmur at the tricuspid area during the routine antenatal visit. She gives history of shortness of breath for the past 2 years while doing more than ordinary work. Which chambers are abnormal based on the ECG?

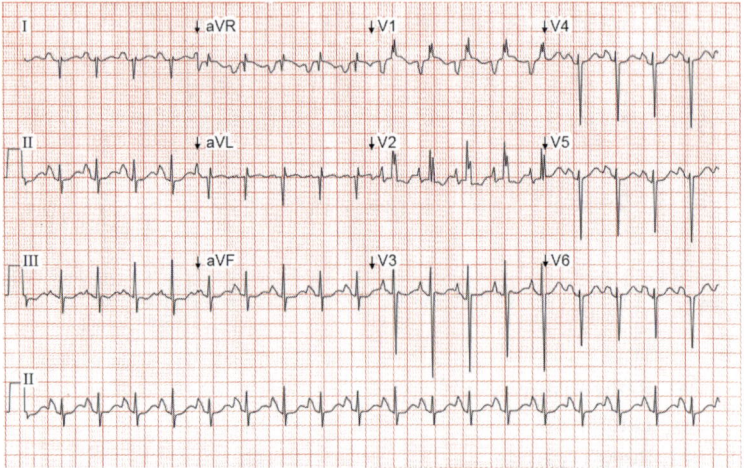

(a) Right and left atria
(b) Right atrium and left ventricle
(c) Left atrium and left ventricle
(d) Right and left ventricles

The ECG shows tall and peaked P waves in lead II and prominent negativity in lead V1. The amplitude of the P wave is more than 2.5 mm in lead II. The negativity is more than 1 mm in depth and width in lead V1. These features are suggestive of both the right and left atrial enlargements. In addition, there is, evidence of the right ventricular enlargement also (R in V1 plus S in V6 >11 mm). The patient has mitral stenosis and tricuspid regurgitation that has resulted in left atrial, right atrial and right ventricular enlargements.

6. A 67-year-old man was seen during routine evaluation for hypertension. He is a chronic smoker and smokes three packs of beedies daily. Which chambers are abnormal based on the ECG?

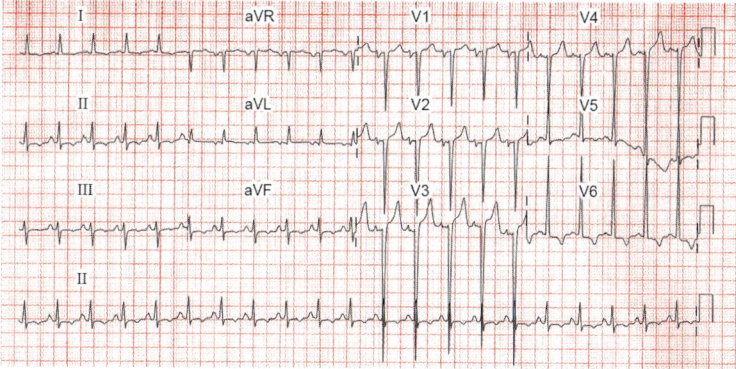

(a) Right and left atrium
(b) Right and left ventricle
(c) Right atrium and left ventricle
(d) Left atrium and left ventricle

The ECG shows deep S waves in leads V1–V4 and prominent R waves in leads V5/V6. These deflections fulfil the criteria for the left ventricular hypertrophy (R wave in V5/V6 >26 mm; S in V1 plus R in V5/V6 >35 mm). In addition, the P waves in lead V1 display prominent negative component that is more than 1 mm in depth and width. This is suggestive of left atrial enlargement. Thus, the patient has combined left atrial and left ventricular enlargements. This combination is frequently seen in patients with hypertension. Systemic hypertension causes pressure overload, which results in left ventricular hypertrophy and left atrial dilatation.

7. A 30-year-old male presented with one episode of syncope. He is asymptomatic otherwise. His elder brother had sudden cardiac death at the age of 35 years. His blood pressure was normal and the pulse showed bisferiens character. Based on the ECG, which chamber of the heart is abnormal?

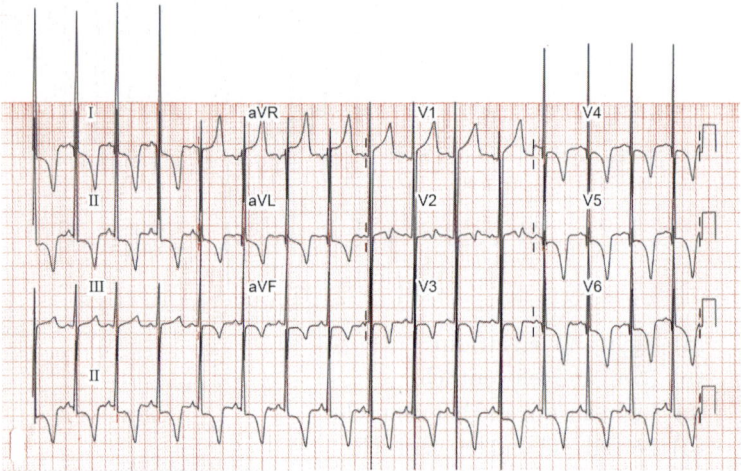

(a) Right atrium
(b) Left atrium
(c) Right ventricle
(d) Left ventricle

The ECG shows tall R waves in inferolateral leads and deep S waves in leads V1/V2. These features satisfy the criteria for the diagnosis of left ventricular hypertrophy. The patient probably has hypertrophic cardiomyopathy based on the history and clinical features. Hypertrophic cardiomyopathy is associated with syncope and sudden cardiac death in the young.

8. A 55-year-old male, known patient of rheumatic heart disease, underwent ECG recording for the evaluation of palpitations. What is the abnormality seen in the ECG?

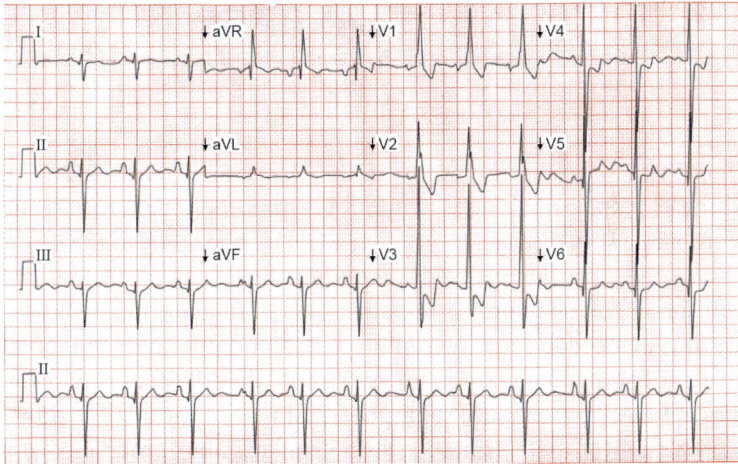

(a) Left ventricular hypertrophy
(b) Right ventricular hypertrophy
(c) Biventricular hypertrophy
(d) No chamber enlargement

The ECG shows features of both right ventricular enlargement (tall R waves in V1 and V2) and left ventricular enlargement (tall R waves in V5). Also there is a large equiphasic complex in V4 suggesting biventricular enlargement.

10   **Coronary Artery Disease**

The ECG has an important role in the diagnosis of coronary artery disease, especially acute coronary syndromes. Atherosclerotic coronary artery disease leads to impaired blood supply to the heart. When the obstruction by the atheromatous plaque is moderate and stable, blood supply is impaired only during exertion, whereas during acute coronary syndrome, the blood supply is impaired at rest. During acute coronary syndrome, there is acute ischemia precipitated by plaque rupture, resulting in subtotal or total obstruction of the coronary artery. Repolarization process is very sensitive to ischemia and is the first to be affected. This is represented in the ECG by ST segment and T wave changes. Very severe degrees of ischemia will affect the depolarization process as well, especially the terminal part.

During moderate ischemia that occurs with exertion, there is ST segment depression. ST segment depression which is horizontal or downsloping and more than 1 mm is significant. The more the number of leads that show ST segment depression, the greater is the extent of ischemia. These changes revert to normal once the exertion is stopped.

When there is ischemia secondary to decreased blood supply as with acute coronary syndromes, a wide variety of changes are produced. Initially, there may be only T wave inversion accompanied by ST depression (unstable angina and non-ST elevation myocardial infarction). Then as the severity of ischemia increases, there will be ST segment elevation and distortion of the terminal part of QRS complex (ST elevation myocardial infarction).

So, in a patient presenting with acute chest pain suggestive of ischemia, unstable angina is diagnosed when there is ST segment depression and T wave inversion. In such a situation, if the cardiac enzymes are elevated (troponins and CPK-MB), then the diagnosis will be non-ST elevation myocardial infarction.

Acute myocardial infarction is diagnosed by coving ST segment elevation in two or more anatomically contiguous leads. The criteria are as mentioned under the ST segment section. The leads showing the ST segment elevation will help us locate the site of myocardial infarction. Leads II, III and aVF represent the inferior wall. Leads I, aVL, V5 and V6 represent the lateral wall. Leads V1-V6 represent the anterior wall, V1-V3 represent anteroseptal wall and V4-V6 anterolateral wall. Leads I and aVL are also called the high lateral wall.

As the MI evolves, there is resolution of the ST segment elevation and development of Q waves with T wave inversion. In the chronic stage, there will be only abnormal Q waves. Sometimes- the patient will present with very severe degree of ischemia and this will be represented in the ECG by decreased amplitude of the R wave, very tall ST segment elevation and tall T waves. This is called the hyperacute phase. In a patient presenting with acute ischemic chest pain, irrespective of whether the ECG shows acute or hyperacute or evolved stage, the importance of the ECG is to diagnose acute myocardial infarction and proceed with timely reperfusion (percutaneous or pharmacological) in the absence of contraindication.

1. A 32-year-old woman complained of pricking precordial chest pain of one-week duration. She has no risk factors for coronary artery disease. What is the ECG suggestive of?

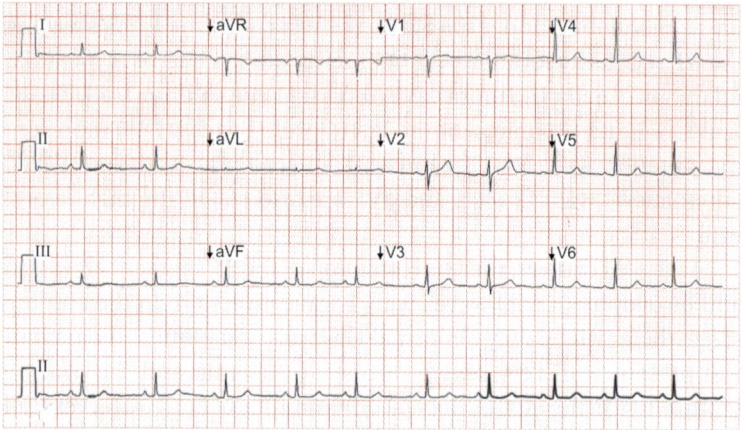

(a) Acute myocardial infarction
(b) Unstable angina
(c) Within normal limits
(d) Pericarditis

Resting ECG shows normal sinus rhythm, normal P, QRS and T waves. The ST segment is normal. Myocardial infarction is characterized by ST segment elevation. In unstable angina, there will be abnormal ST segment depression or T inversion. In pericarditis, there will be ST elevation with PR segment depression in multiple leads. However, in a patient presenting with chest pain, a single normal ECG does not exclude acute coronary syndrome. If the suspicion is high, then serial ECGs are indicated.

2. A 45-year-old man presented to the emergency with retrosternal chest discomfort radiating to the left arm for the past 30 minutes. He smokes two packs of cigarettes per day and is on treatment for hypertension. An ECG was recorded. What is the probable diagnosis?

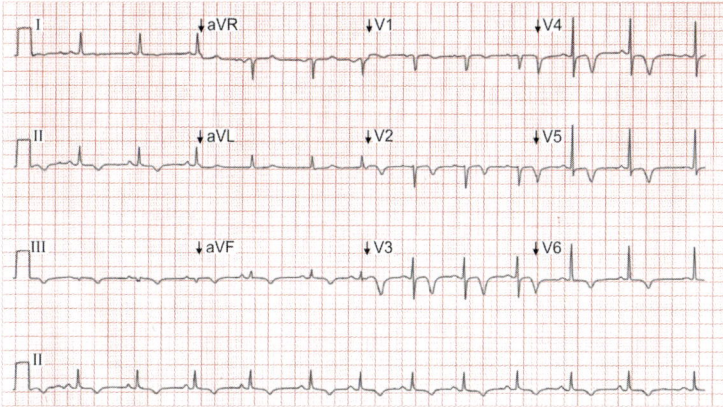

(a) Unstable angina
(b) Chronic stable angina
(c) ST elevation myocardial infarction
(d) Esophageal spasm

The ECG shows significant T inversion in leads V1 to V6 (up to 5 mm) as well as in inferior leads. These ECGs change as well as a history of ongoing rest angina for 30 minutes makes a clinical diagnosis of unstable angina. If cardiac enzymes are found to be elevated, this is diagnosed as non-ST elevation myocardial infarction. In chronic stable angina, resting ECG may be normal.

3. A 57-year-old woman presented to the emergency with history of retrosternal burning pain for the past two hours. The pain was not relieved with antacids. She is on treatment for diabetes mellitus. What is the probable diagnosis based on the ECG?

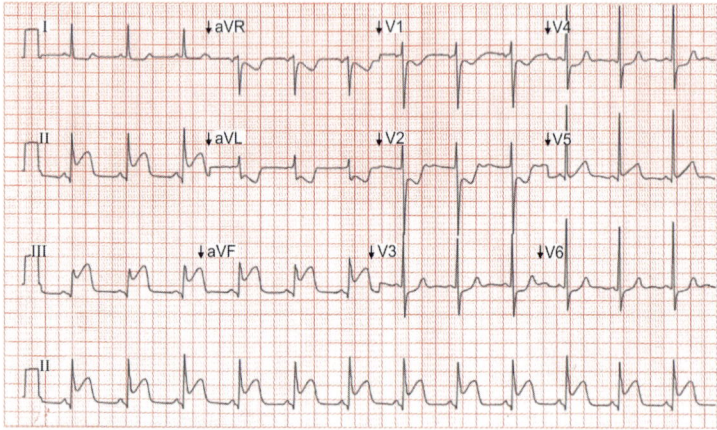

(a) Unstable angina
(b) Gastroesophageal reflux
(c) Acute myocardial infarction
(d) Costochondritis

The ECG shows abnormal ST elevation in leads II, III and aVF. There is ST depression in leads I, aVL, V1–V4. This is suggestive of acute inferior wall ST elevation myocardial infarction. ECG will be normal in gastroesophageal reflux and costochondritis. In unstable angina, there will be ST-T depression and inversion, but not ST elevation. Leads II, III and aVF represent the inferior wall of the left ventricle and, hence, ST elevation in these leads is seen in acute inferior wall myocardial infarction. In anterior wall myocardial infarction, the ST segment will be elevated in anterior leads, i.e. leads V1–V4. In extensive anterior wall myocardial infarction, there will be ST elevation in leads I, aVL, V1–V6.

4. A 52-year-old man complained of severe retrosternal chest discomfort associated with sweating and nausea for the past 30 minutes. What is the finding in the ECG that was recorded?

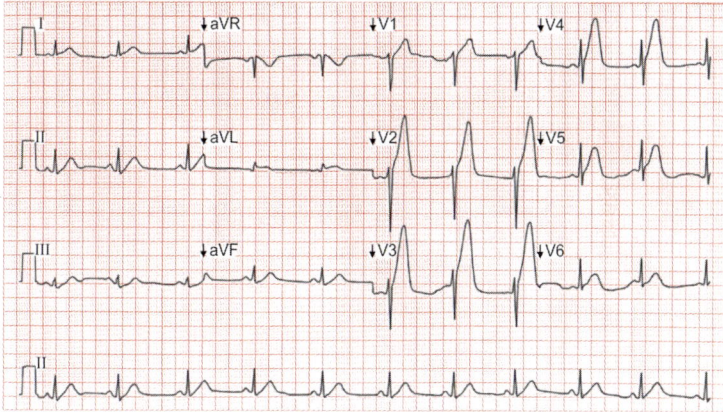

(a) Hyperacute myocardial infarction
(b) Evolved myocardial infarction
(c) Old myocardial infarction
(d) Normal

The notable finding in the ECG is the presence of tall T wave in leads V2–V5. This, along with the presence of severe retrosternal chest discomfort, is suggestive of hyper-acute myocardial infarction. In evolved myocardial infarction, there will be T wave inversion. Old MI is characterized by the presence of abnormal Q wave and the T waves may be normal or inverted.

5. A 45-year-old man was admitted in the ICU for acute myocardial infarction. Where is the infarction located based on the ECG?

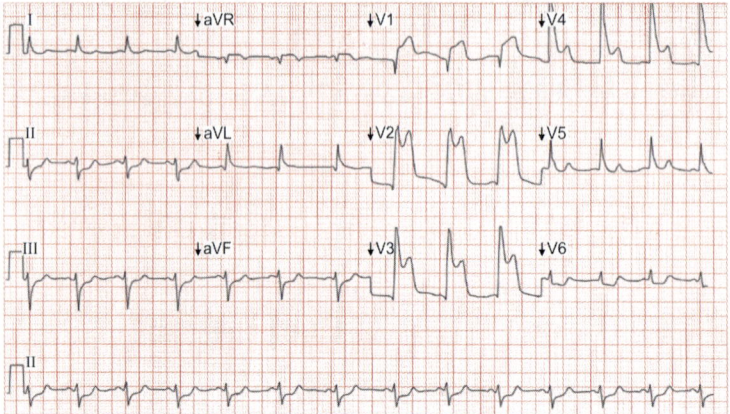

(a) Anterior wall
(b) Inferior wall
(c) Posterior wall
(d) Lateral wall

The ECG shows ST segment elevation in leads V1–V4. In anterior wall ST elevation MI, there will be ST elevation in leads V1–V4. These are the leads that record electrical activity from the anterior wall of the left ventricle. In addition, there may be ST segment elevation in leads V5–V6, I and aVL depending on the extent of infarction. In inferior wall ST elevation MI, there will be ST elevation in leads II, III and aVF. Posterior wall MI is characterized by ST depression and tall positive T wave in leads V1–V2 and ST elevation in posterior leads (V7–V9). In lateral wall MI, there will be ST elevation in leads I, aVL and V5–V6. ST segment elevation has good specificity for localizing the site of infarct. On the other hand, ST segment depression is a poor parameter to localize the site of ischemia or infarct.

6. A 60-year-old woman received thrombolytic treatment for acute myocardial infarction. The 12 lead ECG showed AV wenckebach type of block. Based on the ST elevation, where is the infarction located?

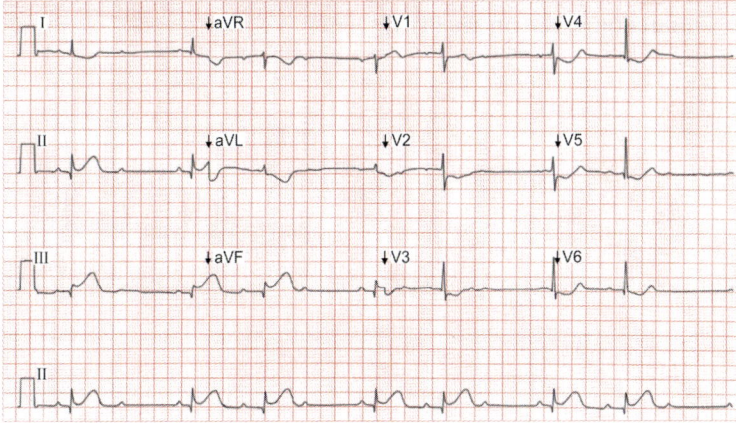

(a) Anterior wall
(b) Inferior wall
(c) Posterior wall
(d) Lateral wall

In this ECG, there is ST segment elevation in leads II, III and aVF. This is suggestive of inferior wall MI. In addition, there is bradycardia and the rhythm is irregular. The PR interval is varying and some of the P waves are not followed by a QRS complex (better appreciated in the rhythm strip at the bottom). There is progressive prolongation of the PR interval until one P waves is not conducted to the ventricle. For every three P waves, there are only two QRS complexes. This pattern is suggestive of type IIa (Wenckebach) AV block with 3:2 conduction. Inferior wall MI is frequently accompanied by AV block, which usually resolves when the MI is treated. Symptomatic patients will require temporary pacemaker support till the conduction becomes normal.

7. A 38-year-old man complained of severe retrosternal chest discomfort radiating to the jaw and left arm for the past 15 minutes. He smokes two packs of cigarettes daily. His elder brother had undergone coronary artery bypass grafting (CABG) surgery for triple vessel disease. Where is the location of the infarction based on the ECG?

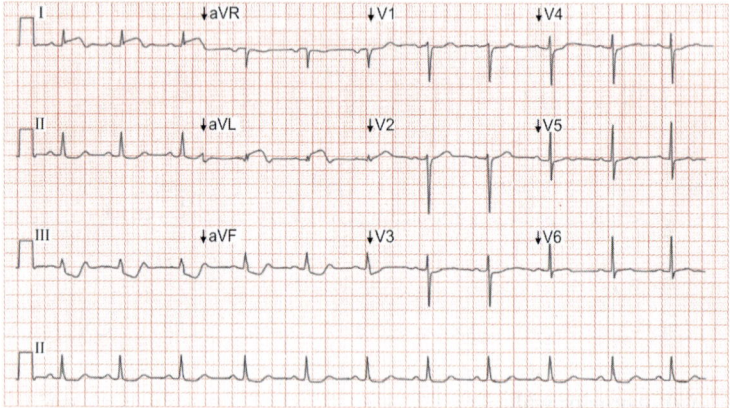

(a) Anterior wall
(b) Inferior wall
(c) Posterior wall
(d) Lateral wall

The ECG shows ST elevation in leads I and aVL. There is ST depression in leads II, III and aVF. This is suggestive of lateral wall myocardial infarction. ST depression in inferior leads is a reciprocal change due to the ST elevation in lateral leads. In anterior wall myocardial infarction, there can be reciprocal changes in the inferior leads and, similarly, in inferior wall myocardial infarction, there can be reciprocal ST depression in anterior leads.

8. A 50-year-old man presented with dyspnea on exertion and gives history of paroxysmal nocturnal dyspnea. He is on treatment for diabetes mellitus for the past 15 years. What does the ECG show?

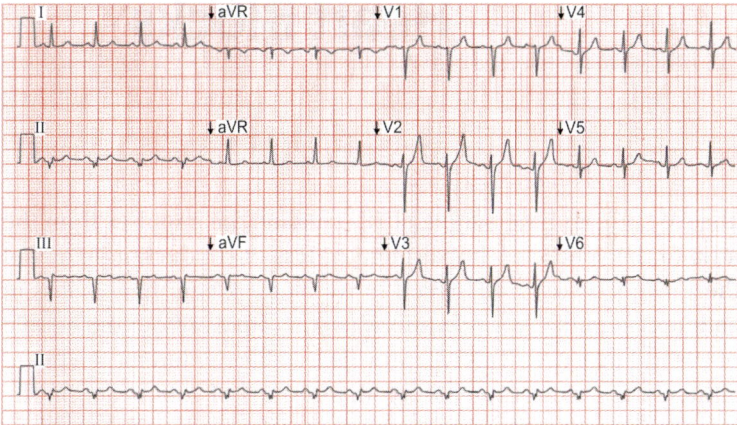

(a) Acute myocardial infarction
(b) Recent myocardial infarction
(c) Old myocardial infarction
(d) Normal

The ECG shows abnormal Q waves in leads II, III and aVF. There is no ST segment elevation/depression or T wave changes. This ECG is suggestive of old inferior wall MI. Presence of Q wave indicates scar in the myocardium. The patient possibly had old myocardial infarction and is now presenting with features of left ventricular dysfunction because of it. Diabetic patients can have infarction without any symptoms (silent myocardial infarction).

11   Heart Blocks

▨ ATRIOVENTRICULAR BLOCK

The AV node and the bundle of His conduct the impulses from the atria to the ventricles. Impairment or loss of conduction in any of these two structures will result in AV block. When there is loss of conduction in the AV node, subsidiary pacemaker from the bundle of His will take over. This will provide a stable rhythm for the heart, although at a slower rate. When there is loss of conduction in the bundle of His, the subsidiary pacemakers from the bundle branches, Purkinje network or ventricular cells take over the rhythm of the heart. But this rhythm is very unstable and can be associated with syncope. Thus, when there is intermittent AV block, it is very important to locate the site of block for prognostication. Based on the degree of conduction block, atrioventricular (AV) block is divided into three degrees.

First Degree Block

In first degree AV block, there is impaired conduction. All the atrial impulses are conducted to the ventricles, but the conduction time is prolonged. This is manifested by a prolonged PR interval in the ECG and one-to-one P-QRS relationship.

Second Degree Block

In second degree AV block, there is intermittent AV conduction; only some of the atrial impulses reach the ventricles while others are blocked. This will lead to an irregular pattern of QRS complexes in the ECG. There are two types of second degree AV block. In type I, there is progressive prolongation of the PR interval with one-to-one AV conduction until one P is not conducted. In type II, the PR interval remains constant, but one or more P waves are not conducted. The number of conducted P waves can vary before the development of block. A 3:2 AV block means that for every three P waves, only two are conducted (two QRS complexes seen). A 5:4 AV block means that for every five P waves, only four are conducted.

Third Degree Block

In third degree AV block, there is loss of conduction from the atria to the ventricles. None of the atrial impulses are conducted to the ventricles. The P waves in the ECG will be dissociated from the QRS complexes. P waves and QRS complexes will have different rates. The classic finding is the marching of P waves through the QRS complex. When the site of block is the AV node, the QRS complexes will be narrow because the escape focus will be in the bundle of His. When the site of block is in the bundle of His, the QRS complexes will be wide because the escape focus will be in the bundle branches, Purkinje fibers or the ventricles.

BUNDLE BRANCH BLOCKS

Block or impaired conduction in one of the bundles will not cause bradycardia per se as the other bundle is available for conducting the impulses from the atria to the ventricles. Bundle branch block will lead to abnormal activation of the ventricles and is identified by the presence of a wide QRS complex in the ECG.

Block in the bundles can be physiologic or pathologic. Pathologic block occurs due to fibrosis of the bundles as seen in many disease conditions like coronary artery disease, systemic hypertension and dilated cardiomyopathy. Physiologic block occurs when the supraventricular impulses reach the bundles before they have completely recovered from the previous depolarization. This happens during tachycardia. When the heart rate normalizes, the bundle branch block resolves. Bundle branch blocks are identified by looking at the QRS morphology in leads V1 and V6 mainly.

Right Bundle Branch Block

The right bundle branch block (RBBB) is identified by the presence of rSR' pattern in lead V1 and deep S waves in lead V6. If the QRS duration is more than 120 ms, it is called complete RBBB. If the QRS duration is less than 120 ms, it is called incomplete RBBB. The QRS axis is usually normal.

Left Bundle Branch Block

The left bundle branch block (LBBB) is identified by the presence of rS or QS pattern in V1 and M pattern or Rs pattern in V6. LBBB is called complete if the QRS duration is more than 120 ms and incomplete if less than 120 ms. The QRS axis in the frontal plane is normal.

■ FASCICULAR BLOCKS

Blocks can occur in the fascicles of the left bundle. Block in the fascicles prolongs the QRS duration only marginally and, hence, the QRS duration can be normal. They are identified by specific patterns of the QRS in limb leads and changes in frontal plane QRS axis.

Left Anterior Fascicular Block

The left anterior fascicular block (LAFB) causes left axis deviation of the QRS. In leads I and aVL, the QRS complexes show a qR pattern and leads II, III and aVF show an rS QRS pattern.

Left Posterior Fascicular Block

The left posterior fascicular block (LPFB) causes right axis deviation of the QRS. In leads I and aVL, the QRS complexes show an rS pattern and leads II, III and aVF show a qR QRS pattern.

Bifascicular and Trifascicular Blocks

To understand this concept, the electrical system of the heart is considered to have three fascicles—the right bundle, left anterior fascicle and left posterior fascicle. LBBB is technically a bifascicular block since it results from conduction block in both the fascicles. The conventional bifascicular block includes RBBB with LAFB or LPFB. It is identified by the combined features of RBBB and fascicular blocks. Trifascicular block means impaired conduction in the third fascicle in association with bifascicular block. A prolonged PR interval in association with bifascicular block will qualify for trifascicular block.

Trifascicular block is also inferred by the presence of alternating bundle branch block. It means all the three fascicles are diseased and they are conducting intermittently. Trifascicular block can be associated with intermittent complete AV block and needs pacemaker implantation.

SINUS PAUSE AND SINOATRIAL BLOCK

Impulses originating from the sinus node reach the atria through the perinodal tissue. Activity of the sinus node is not seen in the ECG. Activity of the SA node is indirectly inferred by the presence of atrial activation in a normal sequence. When there is failure of conduction from SA node to the atria, there will be a sudden pause in the ECG. The duration of the pause will be twice the normal PP interval when one sinus impulse is blocked. There will also be a pause when the sinus node fails to fire in the presence of normal perinodal conduction. However, in this case, the duration of the pause will not be a multiple of the PP interval. Both of these are markers of sinus node disease.

1. A 55-year-old man was seen in the cardiac OPD for hypertension. His medications include metoprolol and hydrochlorothiazide. An ECG was recorded. What is the abnormality?

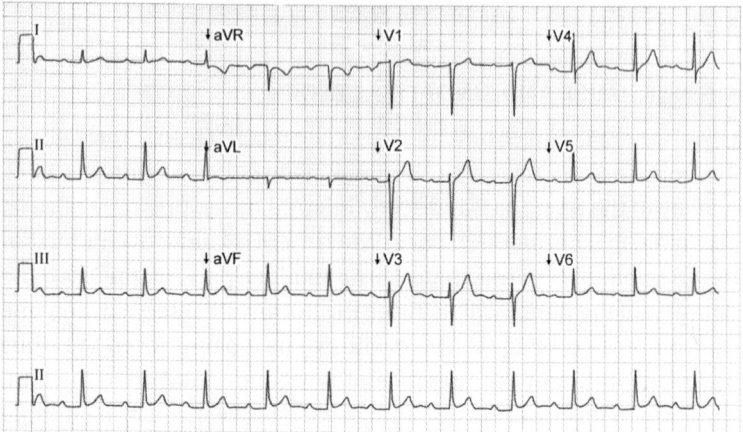

(a) Short PR interval
(b) First degree AV block
(c) Second degree AV block
(d) Third degree AV block

The ECG shows prolonged PR interval. PR interval is more than 200 ms. There is one-to-one relation between the P and QRS complexes. This is suggestive of first degree heart block. Impaired conduction in the AV node or the His-Purkinje system will result in increased time interval between atrial and ventricular activation, manifesting in the ECG as prolonged PR interval. Disease of the AV node, His-Purkinje system and certain drugs can impair AV conduction. Drugs like beta blockers, calcium channel blockers and digoxin can also impair AV conduction.

2. A 34-year-old athlete was noticed to have irregular pulse during routine examination and an ECG was recorded. What is the abnormality?

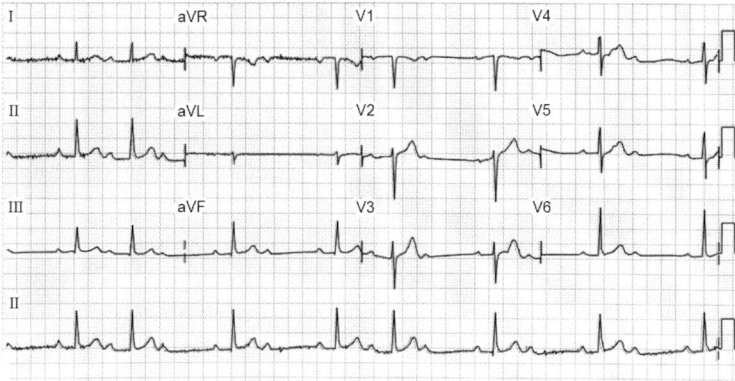

(a) First degree AV block
(b) Type I Second degree AV block
(c) Type II Second degree AV block
(d) Third degree AV block

The ECG shows irregularity of the QRS complexes, best seen in the rhythm strip. The irregularity is caused by episodes of nonconducted P waves. In the sequences where there are two conducted P waves before block, PR interval gradually increases until the nonconducted P wave. This is suggestive of type 1 second degree heart block (Wenckebach phenomenon). Wenckebach phenomenon is characterized by progressive increase in the PR interval, nonconducted P wave and a pause that is less than twice the RR interval. There are two patterns of conduction observed in the ECG: 3:2 (QRS complexes 1, 2 and 4, 5) and 2:1 (QRS complexes 3,6,7). Wenckebach phenomenon is seen when the site of impaired AV conduction is in the AV node.

3. A 45-year-old man was referred for complaints of tiredness. An ECG was taken. What is the abnormality?

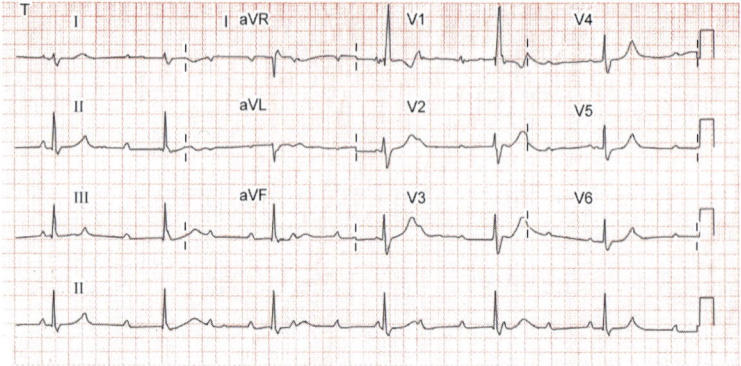

(a) First degree AV block
(b) Second degree AV block
(c) Third degree AV block
(d) High degree AV block

The ECG shows bradycardia with a ventricular rate of about 35 beats per minute. However, there are more P waves seen and these are not related to the ventricular rhythm. None of the P waves is conducted to the ventricle. Hence, this is third degree AV block.

4. A 23-year-old woman was detected to have a cardiac murmur during antenatal check-up. An ECG was recorded and the echocardiogram showed a large atrial septal defect. What is the conduction abnormality observed in the ECG?

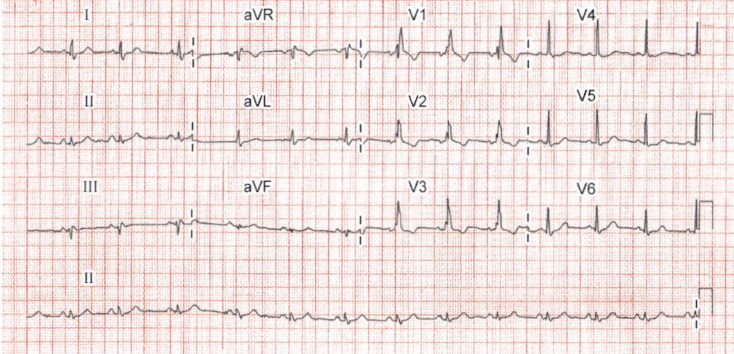

(a) Right bundle branch block
(b) Left bundle branch block
(c) Left anterior hemiblock or fascicular block
(d) Left posterior hemiblock or fascicular block

The ECG shows normal sinus rhythm with wide QRS complex. The QRS pattern in lead V1 shows rsR' pattern. This is suggestive of right bundle branch block. In left bundle branch block, there will be QS or rS pattern in V1. In hemiblocks, the QRS morphology in lead V1 will be normal. Right bundle branch block can be normal or seen in patients with atrial septal defect. Other causes include right ventricular hypertrophy and some congenital heart diseases.

5. A 46-year-old man complained of progressively worsening dyspnea on exertion for the past 8 months. An ECG was recorded and echocardiogram showed severe left ventricular dysfunction. What is the conduction abnormality seen in the ECG?

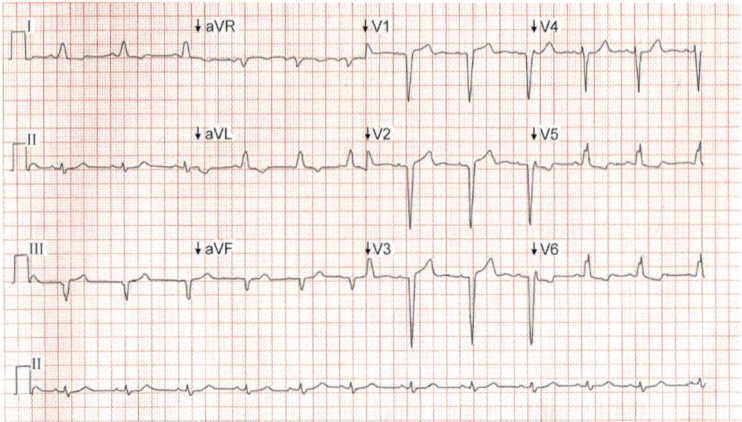

(a) Right bundle branch block
(b) Left bundle branch block
(c) Left anterior hemiblock
(d) Left posterior hemiblock

The ECG shows wide QRS complexes and a QS morphology in lead V1. This is suggestive of left bundle branch block pattern. In right bundle branch block, there will be rsR' pattern in lead V1 and in hemiblocks, the QRS morphology in chest leads will be normal. Left bundle branch can be seen in coronary artery disease, hypertension, dilated cardiomyopathy and in conduction system disease.

6. A 60-year-old man underwent ECG as part of preoperative evaluation for inguinal hernia surgery. The machine-generated report mentioned an abnormal ECG. What is the conduction abnormality seen in the ECG?

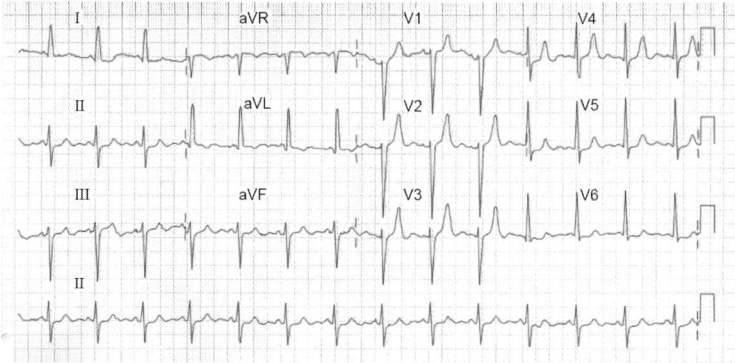

(a) Right bundle branch block
(b) Left bundle branch block
(c) Left anterior hemiblock
(d) Left posterior hemiblock

The ECG shows normal sinus rhythm and left axis deviation. There are qR complexes in lead I and aVL and rS complexes in leads II, III and aVF. The QRS morphology in chest leads appear normal. This is suggestive of left anterior hemiblock.

7. A 52-year-old woman underwent evaluation for pricking left-sided chest pain and neck pain. An ECG was recorded. What is the conduction abnormality observed in the ECG?

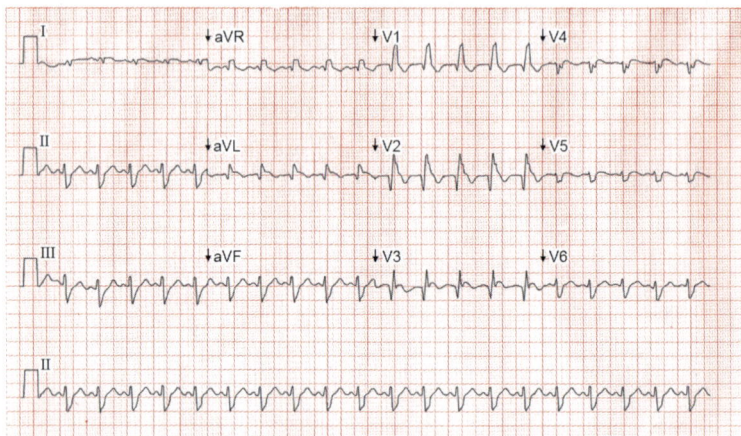

(a) Right bundle branch block
(b) Left bundle branch block
(c) Bifascicular block
(d) Trifascicular block

The ECG shows sinus tachycardia, normal PR interval (120 ms) and a wide QRS with RBBB morphology and left axis deviation. This suggests a combination of right bundle branch block with left anterior fascicular block and is, therefore, an example of bifascicular block. Common causes of this abnormality include coronary artery disease and primary conduction system disease.

8. A 70-year-old man complained of recurrent episodes of syncope. He is a known patient of severe aortic stenosis. What is the conduction abnormality observed in the ECG?

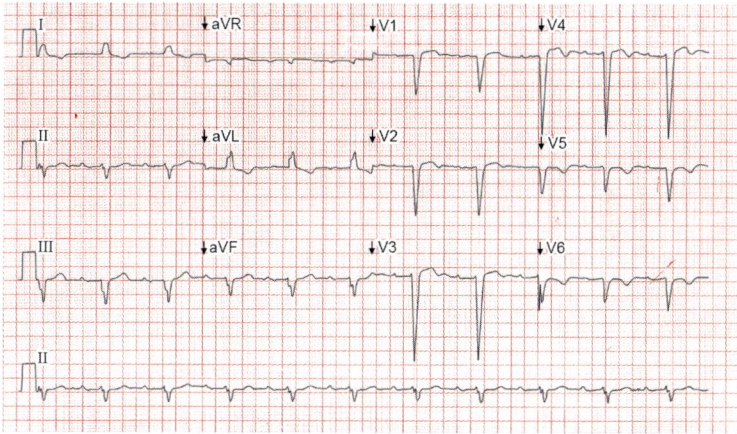

(a) Right bundle branch block
(b) Left bundle branch block
(c) Bifascicular block
(d) Trifascicular block

The ECG shows left bundle branch block (wide complex QRS with QS morphology in lead V1). In addition, there is prolongation of the PR interval. The PR interval measures about 280 ms. This is suggestive of trifascicular block. In this ECG, the left bundle is blocked and in the right bundle, the conduction is impaired, which is manifested as prolonged PR interval. With the history of recurrent syncope and trifascicular block on the ECG, this patient requires pacemaker implantation.

9. A 68-year-old man was detected to have irregular pulse during routine evaluation for hypertension. What is the conduction anomaly seen in the recorded ECG?

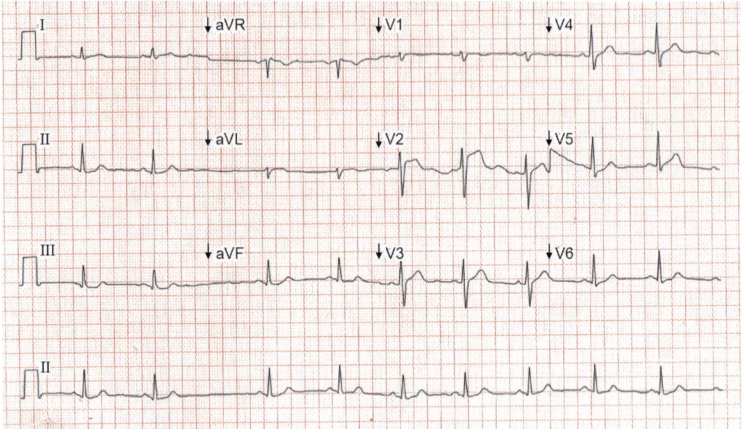

(a) Sinus pause
(b) Sinoatrial exit block
(c) Sinus arrhythmia
(d) Sinus bradycardia

The ECG shows a sudden pause in the rhythm, which is appreciated in the rhythm strip below. Approach to pause in the ECG involves looking at the beats before and after the pause. If there is abnormal beat (early or ectopic) before a pause, then it is likely to be a compensatory pause. If there is abnormal beat (junctional or ventricular beat) after the pause, then it is likely to be pause followed by an escape beat. If the beats are normal both before and after the pause, then it is likely to be a sinus pause. In the ECG shown, the beats preceding and following the pause are normal and so the pause is a sinus pause. Sinus pause is a manifestation of sinus node dysfunction.

10. A 35-year-old man complained of recurrent episodes of presyncope. An ECG was done as part of his evaluation. What is the conduction abnormality observed?

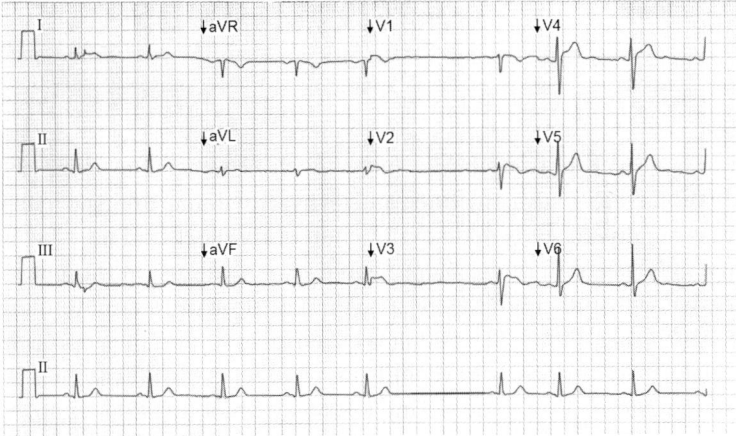

(a) Sinus pause
(b) Sinoatrial exit block
(c) Sinus arrhythmia
(d) Sinus bradycardia

The ECG shows there is a sudden pause in the rhythm and the beats preceding and following the pause are normal. Hence, it is a sinus pause. However, the pause interval is exactly twice the normal PP interval. This is suggestive of sinoatrial exit block. The sinus node fires but because of conduction abnormality in the perinodal tissue, only some of them reach the atria. In sinus pause, the SA node fails to fire regularly, resulting in a pause. Here the pause is usually less than twice the prevailing PP interval. Sinoatrial block is also a manifestation of the sinus node dysfunction.

12   **Arrhythmias**

The approach to arrhythmias begins with classification of the arrhythmia into bradyarrhythmia and tachyarrhythmia. Bradyarrhythmias are due to sinus node dysfunction or AV block and have been already dealt with under blocks and escape rhythms. In this chapter, we will study about tachyarrhythmias. A heart rate more than 100 beats per minute in an adult is called tachycardia. The approach to tachycardia starts with identifying whether the QRS complex is narrow (normal) or wide during the tachycardia. In wide complex tachycardia, the QRS duration is more than 120 ms and in narrow complex tachycardia, the QRS duration will be normal.

NARROW COMPLEX TACHYCARDIA

Narrow complex tachycardia means the ventricles are activated through the normal conduction system by impulses reaching the bundle of His from the AV node and above. That is why they are also called supraventricular tachycardia (SVT). Common SVT include sinus tachycardia, atrial tachycardia, atrioventricular re-entrant tachycardia, atrioventricular nodal re-entrant tachycardia, junctional tachycardia, atrial flutter and atrial fibrillation.

Irregular Rhythm

Next step in the ECG evaluation of SVT is identifying whether the rhythm is regular or irregular. Atrial fibrillation and a type of atrial tachycardia called multifocal atrial tachycardia will cause irregular rhythm. Differentiation between these two depends on the recognition of P wave morphology. In MAT, there will be well-formed P waves but there will be more than three P wave morphologies and there will usually be one-to-one P and QRS relation, i.e. for every

P wave, there will be a QRS complex. In atrial fibrillation, the P waves are not well-formed. There will be constantly varying morphology of P waves with wavy baseline and these are called fibrillatory waves. Sometimes, the P waves are of very low amplitudes and will not be seen in the ECG. Atrial flutter can cause regular rhythm or irregular rhythm. They are identified by the presence of flutter waves. Flutter waves are best seen in lead II and lead V1 and in the presence of irregular rhythm. They have saw tooth pattern without an isoelectric baseline. When there is rapid conduction of flutter to the ventricle (two-to-one or one-to-one), the rhythm will be regular, fast and may not be identifiable.

Regular Rhythm

In the evaluation of regular rhythm SVT identifying the P wave, its morphology and the timing within the RR interval is important. It is not always possible to identify the P waves reliably. Sometimes P waves fall on top of the T wave and will be seen as 'peaked' T waves or they might fall on the ST segment and cause ST-T changes. Carefully scanning all 12 leads especially with simultaneous recording will help in identifying the P wave.

If the P wave is absent, then the diagnosis is AVNRT or junctional tachycardia. If the P waves are inverted in inferior leads, then the diagnosis includes atrial tachycardia, AVNRT and AVRT. When the P waves appear normal (similar to sinus rhythm), then the diagnosis is sinus tachycardia or an atrial tachycardia with focus close to the sinus node. When the P waves are of different morphology from the sinus P waves, then the diagnosis will be atrial tachycardia. If the P waves are inverted in leads I and aVL, then the diagnosis is left atrial tachycardia or left-sided accessory pathway.

Based on the timing of the P wave within the RR interval, regular SVT is divided into short RP (RP interval shorter than PR interval) and long RP (RP interval longer than PR interval) tachycardia. Differential diagnosis of short RP tachycardia includes typical AVNRT, AVRT and atrial tachycardia. Differential diagnosis of long RP tachycardia includes atypical AVNRT and atrial tachycardia.

WIDE COMPLEX TACHYCARDIA

Wide complex tachycardia means the ventricles are activated abnormally during the tachycardia. The differential diagnosis of the wide complex tachycardia is similar to that discussed under wide complex beats. WCT includes ventricular tachycardia, supraventricular tachycardia conducted with bundle branch block, pre-excited tachycardia and in a patient with implanted pacemaker, "pacemaker mediated tachycardia".

Differentiation of the different types of WCT may not be always possible based on the 12 lead ECG. Any WCT in the presence of an underlying heart disease should be treated as ventricular tachycardia unless proved otherwise. However, some ECG findings will help to arrive at a particular diagnosis or support a particular diagnosis. Presence of pacemaker spike preceding each ventricular complex will point towards a paced rhythm. Morphology of the QRS complex during pre-excited tachycardia will conform to specific pathway location. If pre-excitation is present in the sinus rhythm ECG, it will be helpful.

Differentiation of SVT with bundle branch block versus ventricular tachycardia is an interesting topic, but only the very basics will be covered here. VT is favored by the presence of AV dissociation, ventricular capture and fusion beats. Capture beats mean presence of narrow complex beats (sinus beats) during ventricular tachycardia and fusion beat is the fusion of sinus beat and the ventricular beat. Presence of a predominant R-wave in lead aVR is suggestive of ventricular tachycardia. If the sinus rhythm ECG shows a broad QRS, a QRS complex that is relatively narrower in tachycardia is suggestive of ventricular tachycardia.

In SVT with bundle branch block, there will be AV association. The QRS complex morphology will conform to either right bundle branch block or left bundle branch block. If a sinus rhythm ECG is available, it will be helpful to compare the morphology of the QRS complex. The initial part of the QRS will be a sharp and rapid inscription, whereas in VT and pre-excited tachycardia, it will be slow and slurred.

Ventricular Tachycardia

The tachycardia originates from the ventricle and activates the rest of the myocardium. By definition, more than three consecutive ventricular complexes constitute a ventricular tachycardia. It may be divided into sustained or nonsustained. When VT occurs for less than 30 seconds and is hemodynamically stable, it is called nonsustained VT. VT occurring for more than 30 seconds is called sustained VT. There are many causes of ventricular tachycardia and the commonest cause is coronary artery disease.

WPW Syndrome and Pre-excitation

WPW syndrome refers to the presence of pre-excitation in the ECG and recurrent episodes of tachycardia. Presence of an accessory atrioventricular pathway is the hallmark of this syndrome. The pathway can conduct either anterogradely or retrogradely during tachycardia. When the pathway conducts retrogradely, it leads to narrow complex tachycardia (orthodromic tachycardia) and when it conducts anterogradely during tachycardia, it leads to wide complex tachycardia (antidromic tachycardia). Orthodromic tachycardia is more common than antidromic tachycardia.

The accessory pathway connects the atria and ventricles along the atrioventricular groove either in the septum, right or left side. Very minimal pre-excitation may not be obvious in the ECG. Manifest pre-excitation, if present, is helpful to localize the pathway. Presence of a predominantly positive QRS complex in leads V1 and V2 is suggestive of a left sided pathway, while presence of a predominant negative QRS is suggestive of a right-sided pathway. Presence of Q waves in leads II, III and aVF is suggestive of a posteroseptal pathway. More complex algorithms are available to identify the location of the pathway based on the polarity of the delta wave and QRS complex.

1. A 20-year-old woman presented with sudden onset palpitations for the past 2 hours. What does the ECG show?

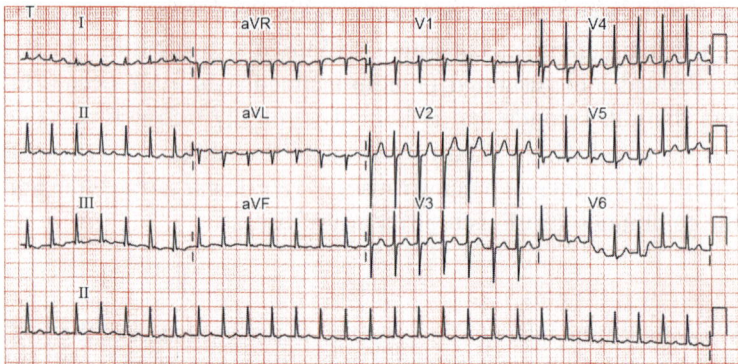

(a) Narrow complex tachycardia
(b) Wide complex tachycardia
(c) Ventricular ectopics
(d) Complete heart block

The ECG shows regular tachycardia and the duration of the QRS complex is normal. This is an example of narrow complex tachycardia. Differential diagnosis of regular narrow complex tachycardia commonly includes AVNRT, AVRT, atrial tachycardia, atrial flutter and sinus tachycardia. P waves are not identifiable in the ECG. This is suggestive of AVNRT.

2. A 32-year-old man presented with sudden onset palpitations for the past one hour. He gives history of similar episodes in the past which used to stop with induced vomiting. What does the ECG show?

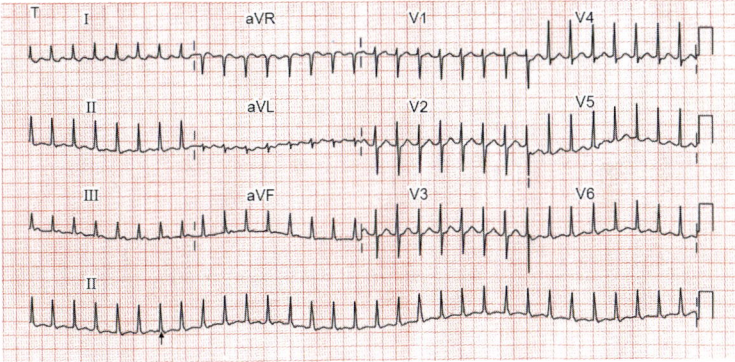

(a) Atrial fibrillation
(b) Ventricular tachycardia
(c) Sinus tachycardia
(d) Supraventricular tachycardia

The ECG shows regular narrow complex tachycardia. In atrial fibrillation, the rhythm will be irregular. In ventricular tachycardia, the QRS complex will be wide (more than 120 ms). Sinus tachycardia will be identified by the presence of normal P waves. In the example shown, P waves could not be identified. Narrow complex tachycardia means that the ventricles are activated from above. Hence, narrow complex tachycardia generally means supraventricular tachycardia.

3. A 65-year-old woman presented with left-sided chest pain of 2 days' duration. She is on regular treatment for hypertension and diabetes mellitus. During evaluation, the pulse was noticed to be fast and irregular. What does the ECG show?

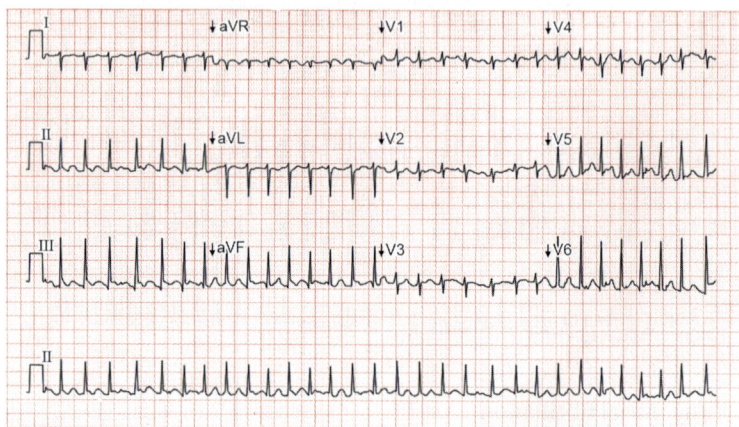

(a) Frequent ventricular ectopics
(b) Atrial fibrillation
(c) Multifocal atrial tachycardia
(d) Second degree type I AV block

The ECG shows a narrow complex tachycardia at a rate of about 180 beats per minute with varying RR intervals. No P waves are seen. This is suggestive of atrial fibrillation. In case of ventricular ectopics, intermittent wide complex beats will be seen in the ECG. Multifocal atrial tachycardia will manifest with P waves of varying morphology. Second degree type I AV block will show progressive increase in PR intervals followed by one blocked P wave.

4. A 50-year-old man presented with sudden onset palpitations of two hours' duration. What does the ECG show?

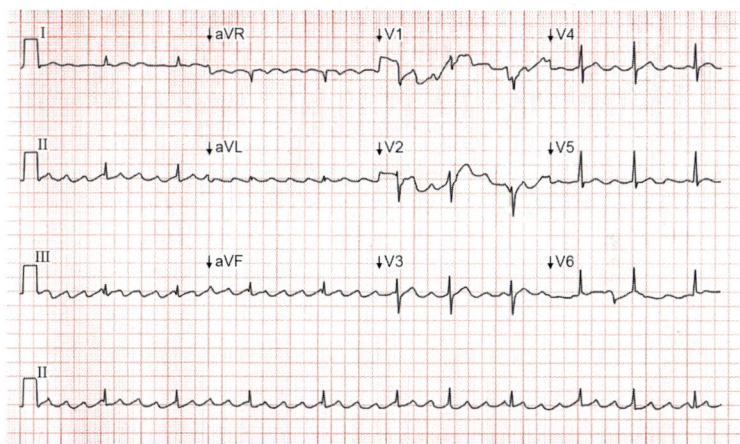

(a) Atrial flutter
(b) Atrial fibrillation
(c) Atrioventricular nodal re-entrant tachycardia (AVNRT)
(d) Atrioventricular re-entrant tachycardia (AVRT)

The ECG shows regular, rapid atrial activity at a rate of 210 beats per minute. The morphology of P waves in the inferior leads resembles a "saw tooth" pattern. This is typical of atrial flutter. The flutter is conducted with a varying AV block and a ventricular rate of about 60 per minute. In atrial fibrillation, regular atrial activity will not be seen. In AVNRT and AVRT, the ECG will show a regular narrow complex tachycardia without typical flutter waves.

5. A 55-year-old man presented with sudden onset palpitations and sweating. He is a known patient of coronary artery disease with moderate left ventricular dysfunction. What does the ECG show?

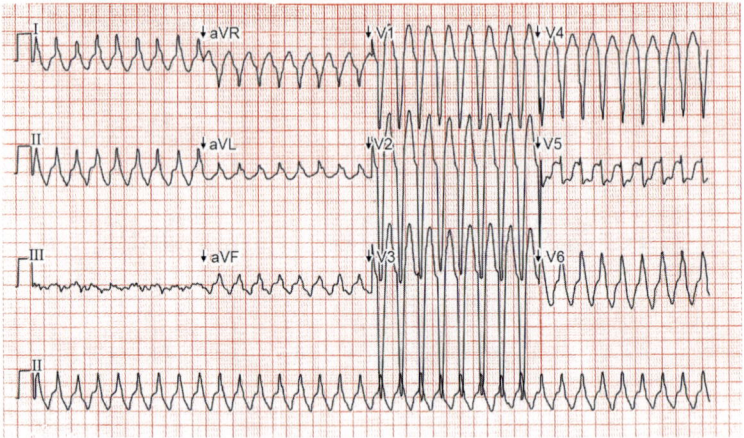

(a) Ventricular tachycardia
(b) Atrial tachycardia
(c) Atrial fibrillation
(d) Artifact

The ECG shows wide complex tachycardia at a rate of 200 beats per minute with an LBBB morphology. Atrial tachycardia and atrial fibrillation will have narrow QRS complexes. Artifact will not show regular pattern. Therefore, the most appropriate diagnosis is ventricular tachycardia, especially in the setting of coronary artery disease and left ventricular dysfunction.

6. A 30-year-old woman was evaluated for episodes of recurrent palpitations. A resting 12 lead ECG was done. What does it show?

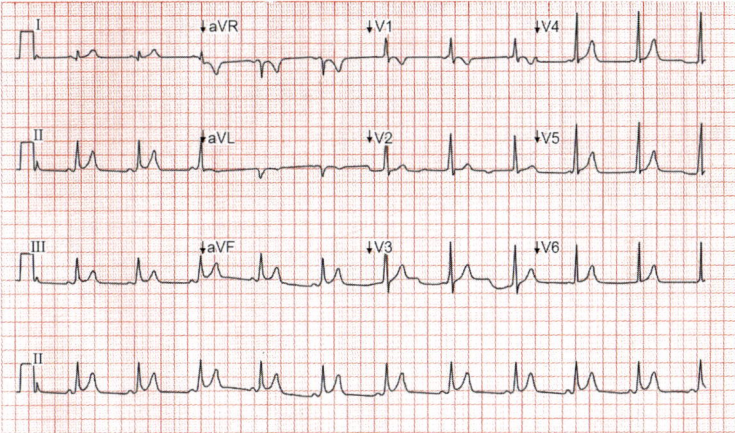

(a) Left-sided accessory pathway
(b) Right-sided accessory pathway
(c) Normal ECG
(d) Acute myocardial infarction

The ECG shows short PR interval and delta wave. The R-wave is dominantly positive in V1 suggestive of a left-sided accessory pathway. The QRS morphology will be predominantly negative in V1 in a right-sided pathway. In acute myocardial infarction, ECG will show ST segment elevation.

7. A 25-year-old man presented with dyspnea and atypical chest pain. What does the ECG show?

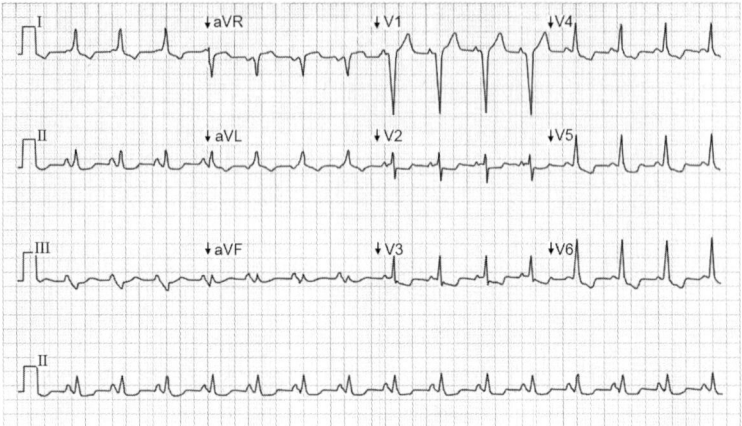

(a) Left-sided pathway
(b) Right-sided pathway
(c) Normal ECG
(d) Pulmonary embolism

The ECG shows a short PR interval and delta waves. The QRS morphology is predominantly negative in lead V1, suggestive of a right-sided accessory pathway. The QRS morphology will be positive in V1 in the left-sided pathway. Pulmonary embolism will show sinus tachycardia and a right bundle branch block pattern in the ECG.

8. A 48-year-old woman was evaluated for recurrent palpitations. The resting 12 lead ECG was normal. ECG during tachycardia is shown. What is the most probable diagnosis?

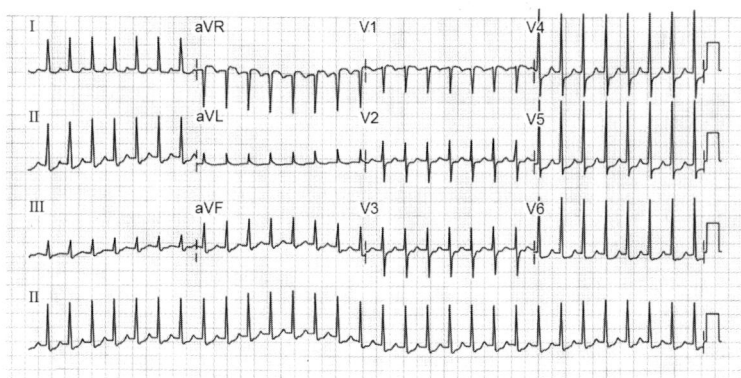

(a) Atrioventricular re-entrant tachycardia
(b) Atrioventricular nodal re-entrant tachycardia
(c) Atrial fibrillation
(d) Atrial flutter

The ECG shows regular, narrow QRS tachycardia at a rate of 180 beats per minute. P waves are seen immediately following the QRS as pseudo S wave in inferior leads and pseudo-r' wave in V1. This is typical of atrioventricular nodal re-entrant tachycardia. In atrioventricular re-entrant tachycardia, the P waves will occur a little later and be seen in the ST segment. In atrial fibrillation, regular atrial activity will be absent and RR interval will be irregular. In atrial flutter, typical flutter waves (saw-tooth pattern) will be seen.

9. A 72-year-old man was admitted in the ICU for respiratory insufficiency. He is a chronic smoker and the present episode was precipitated by chest infection. The ECG monitor showed irregular tachycardia and a 12 lead ECG was obtained. What is the diagnosis?

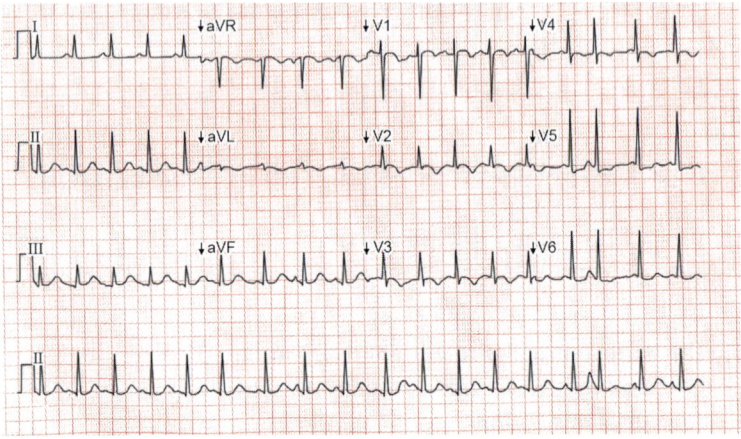

(a) Atrial fibrillation
(b) Multifocal atrial tachycardia
(c) Atrioventricular re-entrant tachycardia
(d) Ventricular tachycardia

The ECG shows narrow complex tachycardia at a rate of about 110 beats per minute and some irregularity of the RR interval. Every QRS is preceded by a P wave and the P wave morphology is varying. The multiple P wave morphologies can be better appreciated in the rhythm strip. This is consistent with multifocal atrial tachycardia. In atrial fibrillation, well-formed atrial activity will not be seen. Atrioventricular re-entrant tachycardia will be regular and P waves will be seen after the QRS. In ventricular tachycardia, the QRS complexes will be wide.

10. A 46-year-old man was admitted to the coronary care unit for acute myocardial infarction and was thrombolyzed. The patient had relief of chest pain, but soon an abnormal rhythm was noticed in the monitor and a 12 lead ECG was recorded. What is the abnormal rhythm?

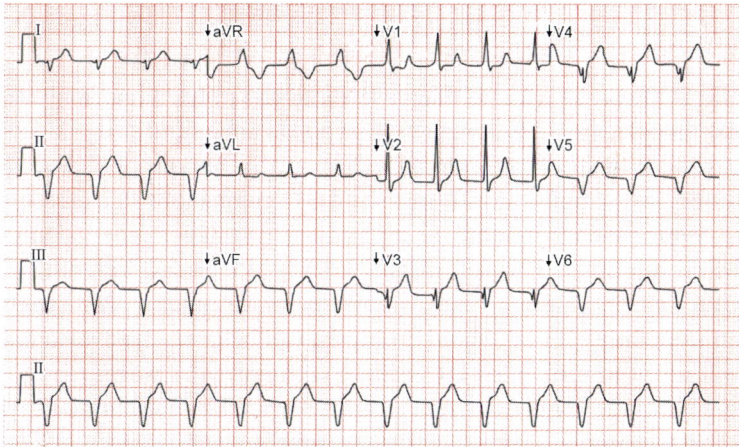

(a) Ventricular tachycardia
(b) Accelerated idioventricular rhythm
(c) Junctional tachycardia
(d) Sinus tachycardia

The ECG shows regular, broad QRS rhythm at a rate of about 80 beats per minute. P waves are not seen. The broad QRS complex suggests ventricular origin, but since the rate is less than 100 beats per minute, this is called accelerated idioventricular rhythm and not ventricular tachycardia. In junctional and sinus tachycardia, the QRS will be narrow.

13   **Miscellaneous Conditions**

The ECG can be used to diagnose some electrolyte abnormalities like hypokalemia, hyperkalemia, hypocalcemia, and drug effects like digitoxicity. Hypokalemia will result in abnormal U waves, diminished amplitude of T waves and QT prolongation. It can result in ventricular premature beats and arrhythmias. Hyperkalemia will result in tall T waves, disappearance of P waves, widening of QRS and, in extreme cases, sinusoidal wave pattern. Potassium abnormalities, if not treated promptly, can be fatal. Hypocalcemia will result in prolonged QT interval with normal T waves. The ST segment is prolonged in hypocalcemia. Hypercalcemia manifests as short QT interval. Digoxin will lead to repolarization abnormalities. It is marked by downsloping ST depression and inverted T waves resembling an inverted tick mark. The QT interval is shortened in digitoxicity. Digitoxicity will lead to ectopics and arrhythmias, usually bradyarrhythmia in children and tachyarrhythmia in adults.

1. A 65-year-old woman presented to the emergency with shortness of breath and decreased urine output for the past one week. She is a known patient of diabetes with diabetic nephropathy. What is the ECG suggestive of?

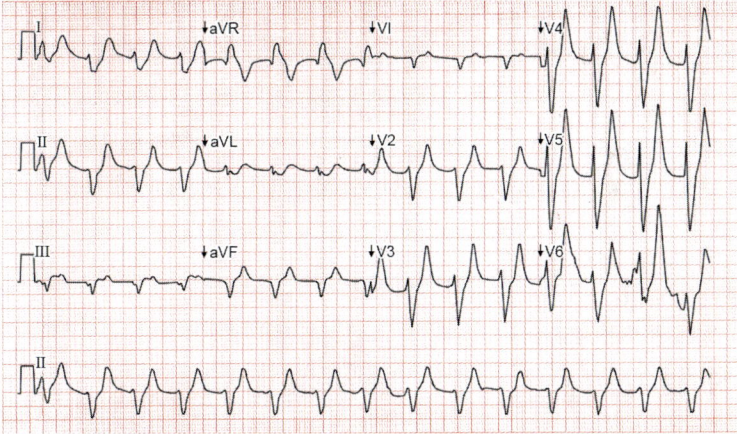

(a) Hypokalemia
(b) Hyperkalemia
(c) Hypocalcemia
(d) Hypercalcemia

Salient features of the ECG include absent P waves, wide QRS complex, and tall T waves. These ECG features are suggestive of hyperkalemia. The clinical history of the patient is also consistent with the ECG. Widening of the QRS is not seen with hypokalemia, hypocalcemia or hypercalcemia.

2. A 35-year-old man was on regular treatment for idiopathic dilated cardiomyopathy. Recently his dose of furosemide was increased for worsening breathlessness. Subsequently, during follow-up clinic visit, an ECG was recorded. What is the ECG suggestive of?

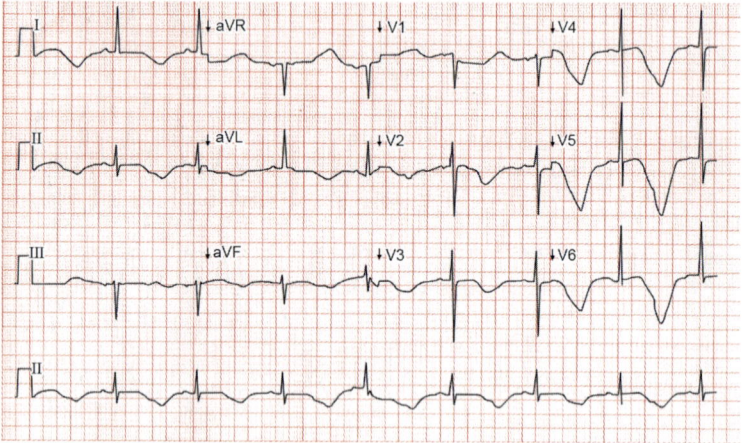

(a) Hypokalemia
(b) Hyperkalemia
(c) Hypocalcemia
(d) Hypercalcemia

The ECG shows deep inverted T waves and a long QT interval. This is suggestive of hypokalemia. Furosemide is a loop diuretic and can cause hypokalemia.

3. A 34-year-old man complained of pricking precordial pain of 3 days' duration. He has no risk factors for coronary artery disease. What is the ECG suggestive of?

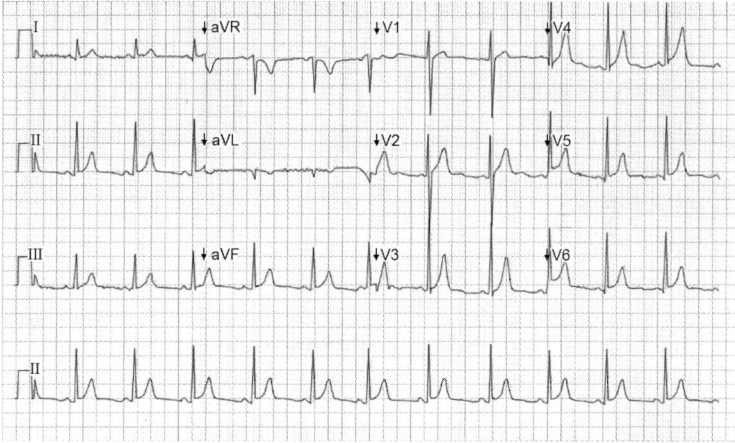

(a) Acute myocardial infarction
(b) Early repolarization syndrome
(c) Unstable angina
(d) Stable angina

The ECG shows normal sinus rhythm, ST elevation in inferior leads which is concave upwards. The ST segment elevation pattern is not suggestive of acute coronary syndrome, where the ST segment elevation will show convex upward pattern. The ECG is suggestive of early repolarization pattern.

4. A 40-year-old male underwent ECG for preoperative evaluation. What does the ECG show?

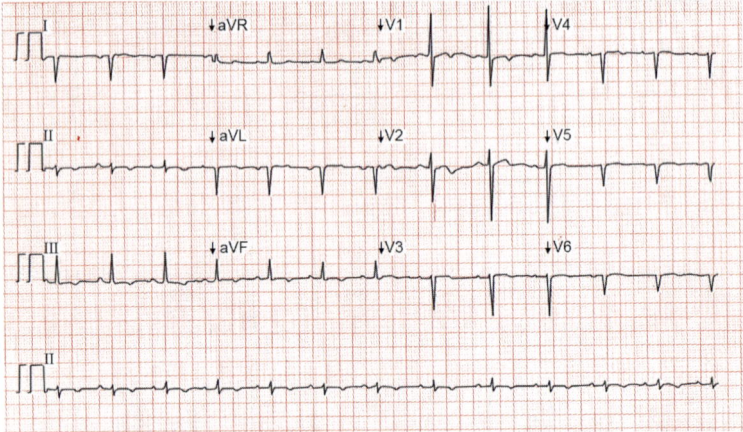

(a) Limb lead reversal
(b) Dextrocardia
(c) Within normal limits
(d) Left ventricular hypertrophy

Salient features of the ECG include inverted P waves in leads I and aVL along with poor progression of the QRS complex in chest leads and QS complexes in leads V4–V6. Inverted P waves in leads I and aVL suggest that the direction of activation of the atria is in the left-to-right direction. This occurs in dextrocardia where the normal sinus node is placed in the left side and activation spreading from it travels in the left-to-right direction. Because the ventricular mass is situated in the right side, the leftward placed leads will record low voltage QS complexes. With LA-RA lead reversal also the P waves will be inverted in leads I and aVL, but the QRS complexes in chest lead will be normal.

5. A 43-year-old man complained of burning epigastric pain and vomiting. He is a patient of peptic ulcer and is on treatment for the same. The attending intern recorded the ECG of the patient and was concerned by the abnormal tracing. What does the ECG show?

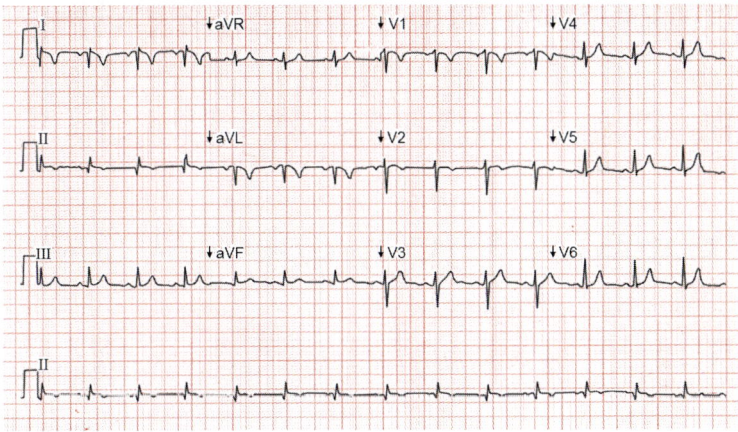

(a) LA-RA lead reversal
(b) Dextrocardia
(c) Ectopic atrial rhythm
(d) Acute myocardial infarction

The ECG shows inverted P waves in lead I and aVL and normal QRS complexes in chest lead.

This is suggestive of reversal of upper limb lead electrodes. The right arm electrode is placed in the left arm and the left arm electrode is placed in the right arm. This will result in the reversal of normal activation pattern and causes the P waves to be inverted in leads I and aVL. This is also called technical dextrocardia.

6. A 30-year-old lady, a known case of rheumatic valvular heart disease, complained of nausea, vomiting and tiredness. Her medications include furosemide, digoxin and oral penicillin. What is the probable diagnosis based on the ECG?

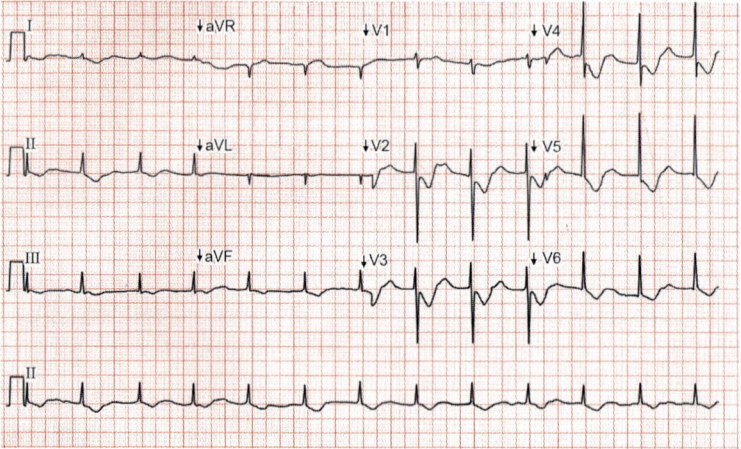

(a) Hypokalemia
(b) Hyperkalemia
(c) Digitoxicity
(d) Within normal limits

The ECG shows accelerated junctional rhythm (narrow complex QRS at the rate of 75 per minute and absent P waves). There is also ST segment depression and T wave inversion in a typical "inverted tick mark" pattern. This, along with the patient's history, is very suggestive of digoxin toxicity. In hyperkalemia, there will be tall T waves and widening of the QRS. In hypokalemia, there will be prominent U waves and prolongation of the QT interval.

Synopsis

▨ BASICS

1. *ECG:* Recording of electrical activity generated by myocardium on a moving graph paper.
2. Graph paper moves at a standard speed of 25 mm/sec.
3. Electrical output from heart standardized to record as 10 mm/mV (amplitude).

▨ LEADS

1. Electrode pairs called leads are used to record electrical activity of heart.
2. *12 leads are used:* 6 limb leads and 6 chest leads.
3. Additional leads are used in special circumstances.

▨ WAVEFOMS

1. Normal ECG consists of waves, intervals and segments
   (a) Waves:
     i. *P wave:* Result of atrial depolarization
     ii. *QRS complex:* Result of ventricular depolarization
     iii. *T wave:* Result of ventricular repolarization
     iv. *U wave:* Result of repolarization of Purkinje fibers and mid-myocardial cells
   (b) Intervals:
     i. *PR:* Represents duration from activation of atria to activation of ventricles (AV conduction)
     ii. *QT and QTc:* Represent duration of ventricular depolarization and repolarization
   (c) Segments:
     i. *PR:* Represents atrial repolarization
     ii. *ST:* Represents initial part of ventricular repolarization

2. Ideal recording should display recordings from all 12 leads simultaneously in 12 rows and a rhythm strip in the thirteenth row.
3. The morphology of the waveforms will vary depending on the lead.

USES

1. Arrhythmias
2. Coronary artery disease
3. Chamber enlargement
4. *Miscellaneous:* electrolyte abnormalities and drug toxicities.

HEART RATE CALCULATION

1. 300 divided by the number of large squares between two consecutive QRS complexes.
2. 1500 divided by the number of small squares between two consecutive QRS complexes.
3. Count the number of QRS complexes in a 6- or 10-second interval and multiply by ten or six respectively (especially for irregular rhythm, use rhythm strip).

P WAVE

1. Look at P wave leads I, II, aVR and V1 (mainly leads II and V1).
2. *Normal P waves:*
    (a) Positive in lead I, II, negative in lead aVR and biphasic in lead V1 with rounded contour
    (b) Positive amplitude less than 2.5 mm in lead II and 1.5 mm in lead V1
    (c) Terminal negative amplitude less than 1 mm in V1
    (d) Duration of P wave less than 2.5 mm in lead II
3. *Abnormal P waves:* Tall, wide, inverted, peaked, notched or absent.

QRS COMPLEX

1. Look at all the 12 leads.
2. Normal QRS complex:
    (a) *Duration:* Between 80 and 100 ms

(b) *Axis:*

    i. *Normal axis:* Predominantly positive QRS in leads I and II

    ii. *Left axis:* Predominantly positive QRS in lead I and negative QRS in lead II

    iii. *Right axis:* Predominantly negative QRS in lead I and positive QRS in lead II

    iv. *Northwest axis:* Predominantly negative QRS in lead I and lead II

(c) *Amplitude:* More than 5 mm in limb leads and more than 10 mm in chest leads.

(d) *Progression:* rS in V1 to Rs in V6, with transition in lead V3–V4.

(e) *Abnormal:*

    i. Wide (duration more than 120 ms)

    ii. Right, left or northwest axis

    iii. Amplitudes less than normal or very tall R waves.

T WAVE

1. Look at all the 12 leads.
2. *Normal T wave:*

    (a) Smooth with asymmetrical limbs

    (b) Direction similar to QRS complex

    (c) *Amplitude:* Less than 5 mm in limb leads and 10 mm in chest leads

    (d) *Duration:* Included in the measurement of QT interval

3. *Abnormal T waves:* Tall, broad, notched, bifid or inverted.

U WAVE

1. Look at all the leads.
2. *Normal U wave:* Positive and less than T wave size.
3. *Abnormal U wave:* Taller than T wave and inverted.

PR INTERVAL

1. Look at all the 12 leads.
2. Measure from P wave onset to QRS complex onset.
3. *Normal:* 120–200 ms.
4. *Abnormal:* Less than 120 ms (short) or more than 200 ms (long).

QT INTERVAL

1. Look at all the 12 leads.
2. Measure from QRS onset to the end of T wave; consider the maximum and minimum values.
3. Correct it for heart rate using the formula—QT interval divided by square root of RR interval in seconds.
4. *Normal:* Corrected QT interval between 450 and 470 ms.
5. *Abnormal:* More than 470 ms.

PR SEGMENT

1. Look at all the 12 leads.
2. Measure from the end of P wave to QRS onset.
3. *Normal:* Isoelectric.
4. *Abnormal:* Elevation or depression (compare with T-P baseline).

ST SEGMENT

1. Look at all the 12 leads.
2. Measure from the end of QRS (J point) to the onset of T wave.
3. *Normal:* Initial isoelectric, gently ascending and merging with T wave.
4. *Abnormal:*
   (a) *Elevation:* More than 1 mm in limb lead and more than 2 mm in chest lead in two or more anatomically contiguous leads.
   (b) *Depression:* More than 1 mm horizontal or downsloping depression in two or more anatomically contiguous leads.

ECTOPIC BEATS

1. Ectopic beats are early beats.
2. Atrial and junctional ectopic beats are called supraventricular ectopic beats.
3. Atrial ectopic beat:
   (a) Normal QRS complex
   (b) Preceded by normal or abnormal P wave
   (c) Normal or long PR interval
   (d) Noncompensatory pause

4. Ventricular ectopic beat:
   (a) Wide QRS complex
   (b) Not related to the preceding P wave
   (c) Compensatory pause
5. Junctional ectopic beat:
   (a) Normal QRS complex
   (b) Not related to the preceding P wave
   (c) Noncompensatory pause.

ESCAPE BEATS AND RHYTHMS

1. Escape beats are preceded by a pause.
2. Escape beats occur due to failure of the ongoing rhythm.
3. Escape beats can be atrial, junctional and ventricular.
4. Escape beat may occur as a single beat or may sustain as a long rhythm.
5. Junctional escape rhythm occurs at a rate between 40 and 60 per minute.
6. Ventricular escape rhythm occurs at a rate less than 40 per minute.
7. *Accelerated junctional rhythm:* Junctional rhythm occurs at a rate between 60 and 100 per minute.
8. *Accelerated ventricular rhythm:* Ventricular rhythm occurs at a rate between 40 and 100 per minute.

WIDE COMPLEX BEATS

1. The differential diagnosis includes ventricular ectopic, pre-excited beat, ventricular paced beat and supraventricular beat conducted with bundle branch block.
2. Pre-excited beats will have a short PR interval and delta waves.
3. Paced ventricular beats will be preceded by a definite pacing spike.
4. Supraventricular beats with bundle branch block will have preceding P waves, initial sharp inscription of QRS and a specific morphology (either right bundle branch or left bundle branch block morphology).
5. Ventricular beats will not be related to the preceding P waves and have monophasic or biphasic complexes.

▩ CHAMBER ENLARGEMENT/HYPERTROPHY

1. Right atrial enlargement:
   (a) Peaked P waves
   (b) P wave more than 2.5 mm in lead II and more than 1.5 mm in lead V1
2. Left atrial enlargement:
   (a) Wide and notched P waves
   (b) P waves more than 2.5 mm in lead II
   (c) Terminal negativity in lead V1 more than 1 mm in depth and duration
3. Right ventricular hypertrophy:
   (a) R wave in lead V1 more than 7 mm or 15 mm (in the presence of RBBB)
   (b) Sum of R in lead V1 and S in lead V6 more than 1.1 mV (11 mm)
   (c) R/S ratio more than 1 in lead V1 and less than 1 in lead V6
4. Left ventricular hypertrophy:
   (a) Sum of S wave in lead V1 and R wave in leads V5 or V6 more than 35 mm
   (b) R wave in lead aVL more than 11 mm
5. *Biatrial enlargement:* Combination of right and left atrial enlargement criteria.
6. *Biventricular enlargement:* Combination of right and left ventricular enlargement criteria.

▩ CORONARY ARTERY DISEASE

1. *Chronic stable angina:* Normal ECG at rest and horizontal or downsloping ST segment depression (more than 1 mm) during stress testing.
2. *Unstable angina:* Horizontal or downsloping ST segment depression with T inversion.
3. *Non-ST elevation myocardial infarction:* Horizontal or downsloping ST depression and T inversion with elevated cardiac enzymes.
4. *ST elevation myocardial infarction:* ST elevation (more than 1 mm in limb leads and 2 mm in chest leads), convex upwards in the corresponding location.

(a) *Inferior wall MI:* ST elevation in II, III and aVF
(b) *Anterior wall MI:* ST elevation in leads V1–V6
(c) *Anteroseptal MI:* ST elevation in leads V1–V4
(d) *Anterolateral MI:* ST elevation in leads V4–V6
(e) *Lateral wall MI:* ST elevation in leads I, aVL, V5 and V6
(f) *Extensive anterior wall MI:* ST elevation in leads V1–V6, I and aVL
(g) *Right ventricular MI:* ST elevation in leads V3R and V4R
(h) *Posterior wall MI:* ST elevation in leads V7–V9, ST depression with tall R in leads V1 and V2
(i) Reciprocal ST depression is seen in leads facing opposite to that showing ST elevation
5. *Hyperacute MI:* ST elevation with tall T waves and distortion of terminal portion of QRS complex.
6. *Evolved MI:* Presence of abnormal Q wave, resolution of ST segment elevation and T wave inversion
7. *Old MI:* Abnormal Q waves, normal ST segment and T wave.
8. *Prinzmetal angina:* ST elevation that settles with or shortly after the resolution of the chest pain.

ARRHYTHMIAS: BRADYARRHYTHMIAS

Atrioventricular Block

1. *First-degree AVB:* Prolonged PR interval
2. *Second-degree AVB:* (Intermittent conduction of P wave)
   a. *Type I:* Gradually increasing PR interval till a nonconducted P wave
   b. *Type II:* Constant PR interval till a nonconducting P wave
3. *Third degree AVB:* (Complete heart block)
   a. Absence of relation between P and QRS
   b. P waves and QRS complexes occur at different rates
4. *High degree AVB:* Two or more consecutive P waves not conducted.

BUNDLE BRANCH AND FASCICULAR BLOCK

1. Right bundle branch block:
   (a) Wide QRS

    (b) rsR' pattern in V1

    (c) rS or RS pattern in V6

    (d) Normal axis or right axis

2. Left bundle branch block:

    (a) Wide QRS

    (b) rS or QS in V1

    (c) M pattern in V6

    (d) Normal axis

3. Left anterior fascicular block:

    (a) Normal QRS duration

    (b) Left axis deviation

    (c) qR in leads I and aVL

    (d) rS in leads II, III and aVF

4. Left posterior fascicular block:

    (a) Normal QRS duration

    (b) Right axis deviation

    (c) qR in leads II, III and aVF

    (d) rS in leads I and aVL

5. Bifascicular block:

    (a) LBBB

    (b) RBBB with LAFB

    (c) RBBB with LPFB

6. Trifascicular block:

    (a) Bifascicular block with prolonged PR interval

    (b) Alternating LBBB and RBBB.

◼ SINUS NODE DISEASE

1. *Sinus pause:* Sudden pause during sinus rhythm and the pause is less than twice the normal rate.

2. *Sinus arrest:* Sudden pause during sinus rhythm and pause is multiple of normal rate.

◼ ARRHYTHMIAS: TACHYARRHYTHMIA

Narrow complex tachycardia: Rate more than 100 per minute and normal duration of QRS.

1. Regular rhythm:

    (a) *P waves absent:* AVNRT and junctional tachycardia

(b) P wave inverted:
   i. *In inferior leads:* AVNRT, orthodromic AVRT, atrial tachycardia, junctional tachycardia
   ii. *In leads I and aVL:* Orthodromic AVRT, left atrial tachycardia
(c) *P waves normal:* Sinus tachycardia, high right atrial tachycardia
(d) *Long RP interval:* Atypical AVNRT and atrial tachycardia
(e) *Short RP interval:* Typical AVNRT, orthodromic AVRT, atrial tachycardia
(f) *Saw-tooth pattern of P waves:* Atrial flutter with fixed conduction (block) pattern to the ventricles

2. Irregular rhythm:
   (a) *P waves absent or not well formed:* Atrial fibrillation
   (b) *Well-formed P waves of more than three morphology:* Multifocal atrial tachycardia
   (c) *Saw-tooth pattern of P waves:* Atrial flutter with varying block.

Wide complex tachycardia: Rate more than 100 per minute and wide QRS complex.

1. Regular rhythm:
   (a) Ventricular tachycardia:
      i. AV dissociation
      ii. Capture and fusion beats
      iii. Monophasic or biphasic QRS complexes
      iv. Concordant or discordant pattern
   (b) SVT with BBB:
      i. AV association
      ii. Triphasic QRS complexes
      iii. Initial rapid inscription of QRS
      iv. Sinus rhythm ECG showing BBB
   (c) Antidromic AVRT:
      i. AV association
      ii. QRS pattern specific to particular pathway location
      iii. Sinus rhythm ECG showing pre-excitation
   (d) Pacemaker mediated tachycardia:
      i. History of dual chamber pacemaker implantation
      ii. Pacemaker spike preceding the P wave

2. Irregular rhythm:
   (a) Atrial fibrillation with conduction down an accessory pathway:
      i. Varying degrees of pre-excitation
      ii. QRS pattern specific to particular pathway location
      iii. Sinus rhythm ECG showing pre-excitation
   (b) Polymorphic VT:
      i. Varying QRS morphology
      ii. Rapid deterioration to ventricular fibrillation.

▮ MISCELLANEOUS

1. *Hypokalemia*: Low amplitude or inverted T waves, prominent U waves and long QT interval.
2. *Hyperkalemia:* Tall T waves, widening of QRS, absent P wave, sine-wave pattern.
3. *Hypokalcemia:* Long QT interval, prolonged ST segment.
4. *Hypercalcemia:* Short QT interval.
5. *Digoxin effect and digitoxicity:* "Inverted tick" ST depression, ventricular ectopics, arrhythmias, short QT interval.
6. *Early repolarization syndrome:* ST elevation in inferior or lateral leads, concave upwards.
7. *Acute pericarditis:* ST elevation in all leads except aVR, PR segment depression.
8. *Dextrocardia:* Leads I and aVL showing negative P waves, early progression of QRS in chest leads.
9. *Technical dextrocardia:* Leads I and aVL showing negative P waves, QR complex and T inversion, normal progression of QRS in chest leads.

15

Appendix

Tachycardia

1. Sinus tachycardia
2. Atrial tachycardia
3. Junctional tachycardia
4. Ventricular tachycardia
5. Atrioventricular re-entrant tachycardia
6. Atrioventricular nodal re-entrant tachycardia
7. Atrial fibrillation
8. Atrial flutter

Bradycardia

1. Atrioventricular blocks
2. Sinus bradycardia
3. Sick sinus syndrome

Tall P Waves

Right atrial enlargement
(a) Tricuspid stenosis
(b) Tricuspid regurgitation
(c) Right ventricular hypertrophy
(d) Pulmonary hypertension
(e) Pulmonary stenosis

Wide P Waves

1. Left atrial enlargement
    (a) Mitral stenosis
    (b) Mitral regurgitation

(c) Left ventricular dysfunction

(d) Left ventricular hypertrophy

2. Intra-atrial conduction defect

Absent P Waves

1. Atrial fibrillation
2. Atrial standstill
3. Junctional rhythm
4. Sinoatrial block
5. Severe hyperkalemia

Inverted P Waves (Leads II, III and aVF)

1. Low atrial rhythm
2. Junctional rhythm
3. Junctional tachycardia
4. AVNRT

Inverted P Waves (Leads I and aVL)

1. Dextrocardia
2. Upper limb lead reversal
3. Left atrial rhythm
4. Left atrial tachycardia
5. AVRT with left-sided accessory pathway

Varying Morphology of P Waves

1. Multifocal atrial tachycardia
2. Atrial ectopics
3. Wandering pacemaker

Wide QRS

1. LBBB
2. RBBB
3. WPW Syndrome
4. Ventricular ectopics
5. Intraventricular conduction delay
6. Paced beats

RBBB

1. ASD
2. Conduction system disease
3. Cardiomyopathies
4. Ebstein's anomaly
5. Brugada syndrome

LBBB

1. Coronary artery disease
2. Cardiomyopathies
3. Hypertensive heart disease
4. Aortic stenosis
5. Conduction system disease

LAHB

1. Conduction system disease
2. Coronary artery disease
3. Cardiomyopathy
4. Congenital heart disease due to endocardial cushion defects

LPHB

1. Conduction system disease
2. Coronary artery disease
3. Cardiomyopathy

Early Progression of QRS

1. RBBB
2. RVH
3. WPW Syndrome
4. Posterior wall infarction
5. HCM
6. Dextrocardia

Late Progression

1. Anterior wall MI
2. LVH

3. LBBB
4. COPD
5. HCM

Left Axis Deviation

1. LAHB
2. Coronary artery disease
3. LBBB
4. LVH
5. Pregnancy
6. Ascites

Right Axis Deviation

1. RVH
2. LPHB
3. Pulmonary embolism
4. Dextrocardia

Northwest/Extreme Axis Deviation

1. VT
2. Endocardial cushion defects
3. Emphysema
4. Hyperkalemia
5. Lead misplacement

Low-Voltage QRS

1. Obesity
2. COPD
3. Pericardial effusion
4. Constrictive pericarditis
5. Pleural effusion
6. Myxoedema
7. Amyloidosis

High-Voltage QRS

1. LVH
2. RVH

3. HCM
4. Thin build

Tall T Waves

1. Hyperacute MI
2. Hyperkalemia
3. Ventricular hypertrophy

Inverted T Waves

1. Myocardial ischemia
2. Myocardial infarction
3. Myocarditis
4. LBBB
5. LVH with strain
6. Juvenile pattern
7. Pericarditis
8. Pulmonary embolism
9. Cardiomyopathy
10. Electrolyte imbalance
11. Subarachnoid hemorrhage

Broad T Waves

1. Raised intracranial pressure, e.g. SAH, ICH.
2. Hypokalemia

Prominent U Waves

1. Hypokalemia
2. ICH

Inverted U Waves

1. Myocardial ischemia

Short PR Interval

1. Accessory pathway
2. Accelerated AV nodal conduction
3. Accelerated junctional rhythm with AV dissociation

Long PR Interval

1. AV nodal disease
2. Digitalis
3. Beta blockers
4. Calcium channel blockers
5. Atrial dilatation

Long QT Interval

1. Drugs:
   (a) Class 1 antiarrhythmics, e.g. disopyramide, procainamide and quinidine
   (b) Class 3 antiarrhythmics, e.g. amiodarone and sotalol
   (c) Tricyclic antidepressants
   (d) Phenothiazines
   (e) Astemizole
   (f) Terfenadine
   (g) Antibiotics, e.g. erythromycin and macrolides
   (h) Antifungal agents
   (i) Pentamidine and chloroquine
2. Congenital long QT syndromes
3. Cerebrovascular accidents, intracranial hemorrhage
4. Electrolyte abnormalities (hypokalemia and hypocalcemia)
5. Physiological—during sleep
6. CHB

Short QT Interval

1. Hypercalcemia
2. Digitalis toxicity
3. Short QT syndrome

Elevated PR Segment

1. Atrial infarction

Depressed PR Segment

1. Atrial ischemia
2. Pericarditis

Elevated ST Segment

1. Acute myocardial infarction
2. Coronary spasm
3. Pericarditis
4. LV aneurysm
5. Myocarditis
6. LBBB
7. Hypertensive heart disease
8. Early repolarization pattern
9. Brugada syndrome

Depressed ST Segment

1. Myocardial ischemia
2. Reciprocal change in acute MI
3. Ventricular hypertrophy with strain pattern

Irregular Rhythm

1. Atrial fibrillation
2. Multifocal atrial tachycardia
3. Atrial flutter with varying AV conduction
4. Ectopics (atrial or ventricular)
5. AV blocks
6. Sinus pause
7. Sinoatrial blocks

Pauses

1. Sinus node dysfunction:
   a. Sinus arrest
   b. Sinus exit block
2. Postectopic
3. Artifact

Early Beat

1. Atrial premature beat
2. Ventricular premature beat
3. Junctional premature beat.

Index